The Legend of Nietzsche's Syphilis

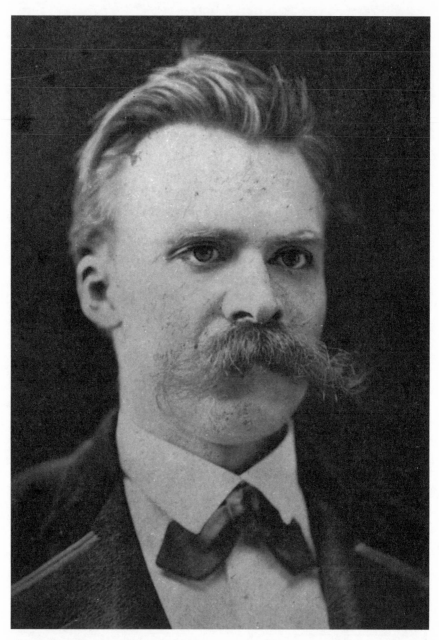

Nietzsche, in 1876, as a university professor. Photo: Stiftung Weimarer Klassik, GSA 101/17; 10–177/167.

The Legend of
Nietzsche's
Syphilis

RICHARD SCHAIN

Contributions in Medical Studies, Number 46

GREENWOOD PRESS
Westport, Connecticut • London

Library of Congress Cataloging-in-Publication Data

Schain, Richard.
    The legend of Nietzsche's syphilis / by Richard Schain.
        p. cm—(Contributions in medical studies, ISSN 0886–8220 ; no. 46)
    Includes bibliographical references and index.
    ISBN 0–313–31940–5 (alk. paper)
        1. Nietzsche, Friedrich Wilhelm, 1844–1900—Mental health.   2. Neurosyphilis—
Patients—Germany—Biography.   I. Title.   II. Series.
    RC201.7.N4 N547   2001
    616.89'0092—dc21   2001023341
    [B]

British Library Cataloguing in Publication Data is available.

Library of Congress Catalog Card Number: 2001023341
ISBN: 0–313–31940–5
ISSN: 0886–8220

First published in 2001

Greenwood Press, 88 Post Road West, Westport, CT 06881
An imprint of Greenwood Publishing Group, Inc.
www.greenwood.com

Printed in the United States of America

The paper used in this book complies with the
Permanent Paper Standard issued by the National
Information Standards Organization (Z39.48–1984).

10 9 8 7 6 5 4 3 2 1

Copyright Acknowledgment

The author and publisher gratefully acknowledge The Goethe and Schiller Archives for
use of the photographs.

To Melanie
mein tanzenden Stern

Contents

Photo essay follows page xv.

Preface

"Yet another book on Nietzsche?" is the phrase with which An-acleto Verrecchia began his controversial 1976 work titled *Nietz-sche's Catastrophe at Turin*.[1] This phrase was actually taken from an earlier Italian book on Nietzsche published in 1902. A century later, the torrent of Nietzsche literature beginning in the last de-cade of the nineteenth century shows no sign of subsiding; if any-thing, it appears to be increasing, since Nietzsche has now become a favorite topic in the English book trade which was not the case earlier. A computer check of the decade 1988–1998 reveals 261 English language books published about Friedrich Nietzsche, the struggling German expatriate whose adult life seemed to be a con-tinual exercise in overcoming suffering and isolation.

Nietzsche began a promising career at 24 years of age with an appointment as a full professor of classical philology at the Uni-versity of Basel. Ten years later, burned out as a faculty person and suffering with a multitude of physical complaints, he resigned his professorship and embarked on a peripatetic life as an inde-pendent philosopher. During this period he produced the remark-able literary opus that was to make him famous. At age 45 he suffered a complete nervous breakdown, which ended his creative life and from which he never recovered. Total dependency and slow deterioration marked the last eleven years of his life. The worldwide fame of his writings developed at this time when he was incapable of relating to anyone around him in a meaningful way.

Whatever one may think of Nietzsche's life or writings, there can be no doubt that he is a major cultural icon at the turn of the twentieth century. The author of the *Untimely Meditations* seems to be perennially timely, reminding the literate world about the necessity for creating one's self. His star temporarily dimmed outside of Germany during the National Socialist era because of the unmerited association of his name with Nazi ideology; but he has since rebounded even more strongly and is now a world figure as compared to his earlier, largely European status. A casual visit to bookstores in the United States will reveal more books on the shelves devoted to Nietzsche than other philosophical or religious authors. There is a level of attention paid to Nietzsche, which cannot be easily matched by any other literary figure.

The interest in Nietzsche is, of course, founded on his writings, which may be regarded as some of the most remarkable productions of Western literature. There is general agreement among critics that Nietzsche was a prose stylist of the first order, whatever one may think of the ideas that he put forth. On this latter question, there is a great diversity of opinion ranging from the many eminent figures who believe Nietzsche was one of the great thinkers of all time to the opinion expressed by Verrechia in his preface that interest in Nietzsche is a sickness in itself. The fact that Nietzsche's life culminated in insanity did not and has not reduced the interest in his writings; in fact, it is likely that his horrible end stimulated this interest.

More than any other category of writer, interest in the thoughts of a philosopher necessarily requires some knowledge of the life from whence these thoughts arose. How could one imagine, for example, that the writings of Spinoza, Schopenhauer, or Emerson could be fully grasped in the absence of any information about their lives. In the case of Nietzsche who wrote at length about himself, it is possible to learn much about him from his writings alone. If one is capable of reading all that Nietzsche wrote; the works published in his lifetime, his letters and his notebooks—all of which are now available in published form—his life would emerge in considerable detail. His biographers have added a wealth of information about the external circumstances affecting him. However, there is one subject which, although widely discussed in the first part of this century in German language publications, has received little attention since the Second World War. This is the matter of Nietzsche's presumed syphilis and its relationship to his mental breakdown.

The question of the origin of the insanity which suddenly came upon Nietzsche, age 44 years, during the first days of 1889, was decided by his physicians to be due to "general paresis," a condition which then was increasingly attributed to syphilis of the brain. This diagnosis was not known to the general public during the decade of the 1890s when Nietzsche, totally psychotic at the time, became a European celebrity. However in 1902, Paul Möbius, a German neurologist and a literary figure in his own right, published a work titled *Nietzsche's Pathology* which revealed the medical diagnosis.[2] Henceforth, a flood of medical and lay literature emerged to argue the merits of the diagnosis and its possible impact on Nietzsche's writings. Most German medical writers who have written on the subject have concurred with the opinion of Nietzsche's physicians. Volz, who has provided the most recent and most comprehensive review of all aspects of Nietzsche's illnesses, concluded that Nietzsche did in fact suffer from general paresis, that is, syphilis of the brain.[3]

The importance of this question to those who are interested in Friedrich Nietzsche can hardly be overemphasized. There are many who prefer to ignore the subject, believing that Nietzsche's creative genius was one thing, his physical self with its illnesses was another and that it is unnecessary to relate the two. This may be viewed as a contemporary manifestation of the venerable mind-body separation which is still present today. However, given that all thought occurs in the context of a functioning brain, it is self-evident that if Nietzsche's brain were infested with spirochetes, it would function differently than if it were not so contaminated. Nietzsche with syphilitic brain disease is a different personality than a non-syphilitic Nietzsche, albeit one suffering with eyestrain, headaches, and severe adjustment problems to the modern world. One needs to know the facts about the status of the brain in an individual who occupies a unique position in the history of Western thought. Whatever one may think about Nietzsche's personality or habits, it is his brain-mediated thoughts which count, the explosive thoughts which finally made him famous. As Henry David Thoreau expressed it in a letter to H.G.O. Blake, "Our thoughts are the epochs in our lives; all else is but a journal of the winds that blew while we were here."[4] This is perhaps more applicable to Friedrich Nietzsche than to any other personality who has impacted Western culture. Parenthetically, it should be noted that there are many similarities in the lives and thoughts of Thoreau and Nietzsche.

This writing concentrates on the medical and psychiatric aspects of Nietzsche's life, specifically focusing on the question of the nature of his mental collapse. Other biographical data are provided to the extent necessary for providing a supportive picture of his life's circumstances. The contention set forth is that the diagnosis of general paresis in Nietzsche is not tenable. This conclusion is based on an analysis of the historical information and current concepts of general paresis as well as the specifics of Nietzsche's mental disturbance and neurological status. Much has become known about general paresis—"*progressive paralyse*" in German medical literature—which was not known at the time of Nietzsche's illness and during the years when the controversy was at its height. Volz provides invaluable documentation on the subject of Nietzsche's illnesses but her discussion is insufficiently critical, at least as far as the diagnosis of general paresis is concerned. It may have been an exaggeration when Verrechia commented on this subject that "an inventive mind sets a suspicion in motion and a thousand '*Dummköpfe*' endlessly repeat it."[5] Nevertheless, it seems strange that a diagnosis based on such flimsy evidence should have been so tenacious in its hold on literary public opinion. It is a legend that needs to be set at rest in order for Nietzsche's legacy to find its proper place.

The *Kritische Studienausgabe* series edited by Giorgio Colli and Mazzino Montinari (Berlin: de Gruyter, 1967 onwards) has become the definitive source of Nietzsche's writings, including his published works, his letters, and his notebooks. However, because of the existence of so many versions of Nietzsche's writings, I have chosen to make reference to the published works by their original title. The letter *s.* refers to the section number containing the relevant quotation which is uniform in most versions. In this way, readers can easily locate the quoted material in whatever form in which Nietzsche's writings are available to them. Nietzsche's letters are identified by the date as given in the *Kritische Studienaus-*

gabe, Samtliche Briefe. Unless otherwise specified, the translations are all my own from the de Gruyter series. My emphasis has been on trying to convey Nietzsche's style rather than on providing flawless English.

Acknowledgments

This work could not have been completed without the availability of the library facilities at the University of California, Berkeley, for which I am grateful. I wish specifically to thank Richard Stach, assistant librarian at the Sonoma Developmental Center for his unfailing assistance. Most of all, I want to acknowledge the role of my wife, Dr. Melanie Dreisbach. Her support and participation were an essential feature of the project.

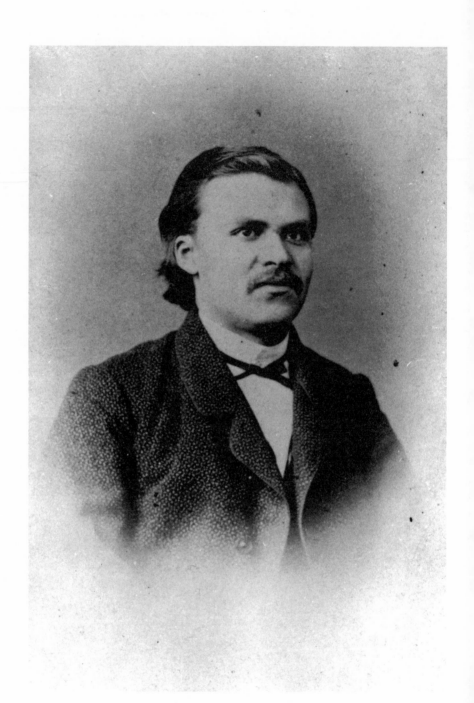

Nietzsche as a university student. Photo: Stiftung Weimarer Klassik, GSA 101/7; 10–168/152.

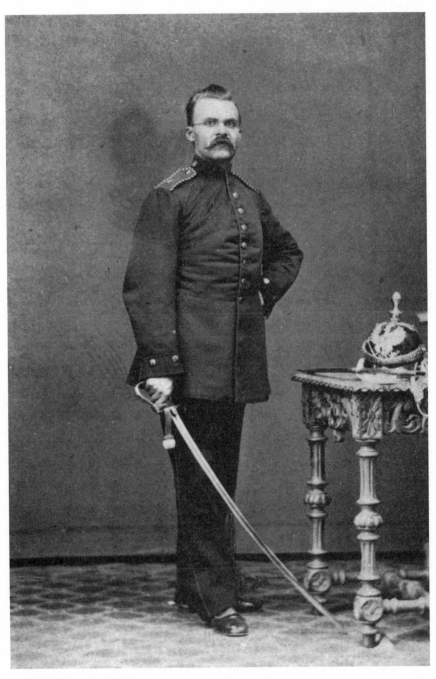

Nietzsche in 1868 as an artillery officer. Photo: Stiftung Weimarer Klassik, GSA 101/9; 10–138/152.

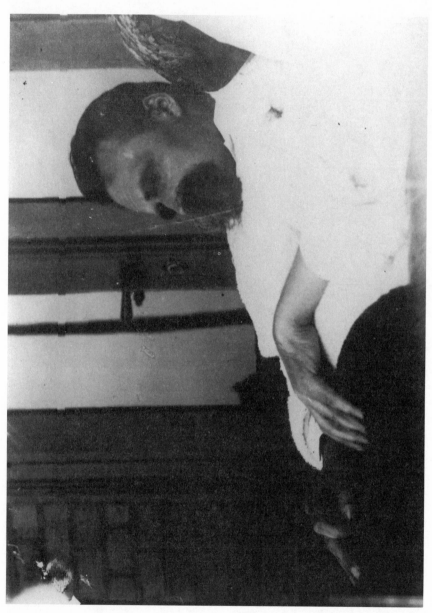

Nietzsche in 1899, totally incapacitated. Photo: Stiftung Weimarer Klassik, GSA 101/37; 10–152/53.

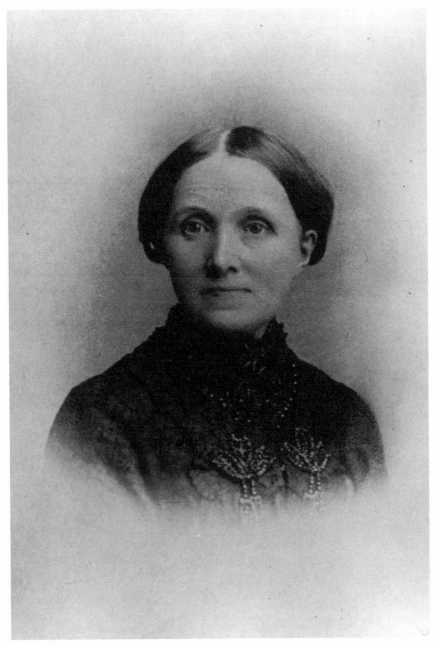

Nietzsche's mother in 1892. Photo: Stiftung Weimarer Klassik, GSA 101/318; 10–138/149.

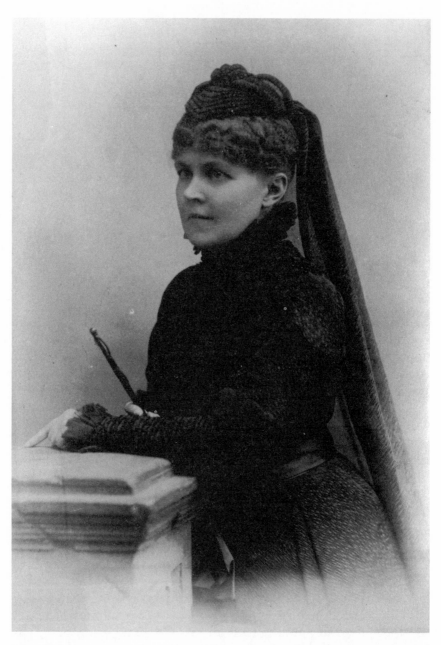

Nietzsche's sister in 1901. Photo: Stiftung Weimarer Klassik, GSA 101/162; 10–47/107.

1

Background

The antecedents of Friedrich Nietzsche (1844–1900) derived from the province of Saxony, a region that had been annexed by Prussia after the Napoleonic era. It was an area dominated by rural, conservative, and Lutheran values. Nothing in the annals of his immediate forebears gives any hint of the meteoric life and revolutionary writings that were to characterize Nietzsche.[1] This may account, at least in part, for the fact that Nietzsche's mother did not have the slightest appreciation of her son's works. His sister, Elisabeth, while founding the Nietzsche Archives and guarding his memory for 40 years, never could penetrate her brother's worldview. Rudolph Steiner, whom she engaged in 1896 to teach her philosophy, deemed Elisabeth completely incapable of understanding Nietzsche's conceptions.[2] This situation is only one of the many paradoxes surrounding his life and influence.

The most important fact about Nietzsche's ancestry is that it contained numerous Protestant clergymen on both parental sides. His later comment that "The Protestant pastor is the grandfather of German philosophy . . ." (The Antichrist, s. 10) applied to himself more than to any other prominent German philosopher. His father, Karl Ludwig Nietzsche (1813–1849), was the pastor of the German Evangelical Church (Lutheran) at the small town of Röcken in the then Prussian province of Saxony where Nietzsche was born. Karl Ludwig's father, Friedrich August Nietzsche (1756–1826), had been an archdeacon in the nearby town of Eilenberg. Members of this side of his family had been pastors for many generations extending back to the beginning of the seventeenth century. On Nietzsche's mother's side, the maternal grandfather, David Ernst Oehler (1787–1859), was a longtime pastor in the town of Pobles. At least two of his uncles on the mother's side were pastors as well. One of them, Theodor Oehler, was later to end his life by suicide.

This clerical genealogy makes evident the truth of Janz's assertion that "The evangelical parsonage was the inheritance which formed Nietzsche's character and decisively determined his early development."[3] Yet the adult Nietzsche publicly and impassionately repudiated his entire spiritual ancestry, an event that probably had more to do with his later mental state than the better known circumstances of his departure from academia or his separation from Wagner. Nietzsche's sister Elisabeth, who assumed control of his literary estate shortly before his death, disseminated the idea that the Nietzsche family came from healthy stock (in conjunction with her assertions that her brother's breakdown originated from overwork and overuse of sleeping pills) but this was not at all the case. Nietzsche's father suffered from a mysterious illness that caused his death in his 36th year of life. He was said to have suffered from "migraine-like" headaches and a year or so before his death he began to exhibit nervous instability with onset of "attacks" of an indeterminate nature which caused him to require assistance with his pastoral duties. At times, he exhibited what appeared to be brief epileptic seizures. Increasing head pain, vomiting, and prostration developed causing him to be finally confined to his bed. Supposedly he became blind shortly before his death.

Unlike the case with Nietzsche, postmortem examination of the father was performed. A "brain softening" was discovered which occupied one quarter of the brain. Another report mentions a brain "tumor" (*Geschwulst*) as having been present.[4] It is impossible to determine the nature of Karl Ludwig's brain lesion from the available information. A true brain tumor may have been present as was believed by Paul Möbius, a prominent neurologist who first publicly discussed Nietzsche's family history,[5] but other possibilities also exist. Some type of vascular malformation looking like a tumor would be more in accord with the rapid progress of symptoms. Other conditions that might produce such a brain lesion are tuberculosis (tuberculomas of the brain were common in Europe at the time) or slow bleeding into the brain occasioned by a head injury. Nietzche's mother claimed her husband's illness was caused by a fall on stone steps but this has been discounted by later analysis of the sequence of events. His symptoms preceded the fall and it is more likely that the episode was a consequence rather than a cause of his illness. However, all these speculations made long after the relevant events are unverifiable.

There is a certain resemblance of Nietzsche's later symptoms with those of his father, although the tempo of the illnesses and final outcome were different. Nietzsche himself believed that his undiagnosed physical problems were related to those of his father and he expected to die at the same age. In the late 1870s, he repeatedly stated he expected a stroke to carry him off. It was at this time that he was forced to resign his professorship. However, other than migraine, which is usually not a life threatening illness, there are no clear-cut genetic factors involved in the various brain disorders mentioned above.

The family physical problems that Nietzsche was definitely heir to are migraine and myopia. As mentioned, his father had recurrent headaches which Möbius thought to be migrainous in nature. One of his father's sisters had a similar problem as did Nietzsche's own sister who could be confined to bed for up to three days because of headaches. The myopia (shortsightedness) which plagued Nietzsche all his life was also an inheritance from his father and affected Elisabeth as well, although she refused to wear glasses.

A third male sibling was born to the Nietzsche family in February 1848 at a time when the father was already showing signs of the illness that led to his death. This brother, Joseph, died at 22 months of age after manifesting seizures (*Krämpfe*) and a terminal "stroke." Not much can be said about the relationship of this illness to the problems of the rest of the family but it is another piece of evidence that the Nietzsche family was indeed affected by a predisposition to neurological disorders.

The Oehlers, Nietzsche's mother's side of the family, contributed a significant number of examples of psychiatric problems to the family constellation. An uncle of Nietzsche's, Theobald Oehler, committed suicide as mentioned above. He had been a pastor in a country town but other details are not available. Nietzsche, in correspondence with his mother on the subject, suggested Theobald had preferred death to the *Irrenhaus*—the nineteenth century German term for lunatic asylum.[6] There is something ironic about Nietzsche's comment; he himself did not make the same choice. Möbius mentions "a number" of the mother's sisters were "mentally abnormal," one of whom committed suicide and another went mad (there were ten siblings of the Frau Pastor Nietzsche-Oehler). The mother herself stated one of her sisters had died in a psychiatric hospital. Finally, in 1901, an 87-year-old surviving brother of the mother developed some kind of mental illness requiring psychiatric care. Much of this information is vague but suggests that Nietzsche's own mental breakdown was nothing unusual within the Nietzsche-Oehler extended family.

2

Early Years

Nietzsche's birth on October 15, 1844, to his eighteen-year-old mother, Franciska, was completely uneventful. He was a healthy, well-formed newborn without congenital stigmata of any type. His early development was quite regular except for some delay in his speech that caused concern to the family. However, by two years of age he was speaking freely, dissipating that concern. No significant illnesses appeared to have occurred during his early childhood.

Young "Fritz" grew up in a typical country parsonage. His sister Elisabeth (1846–1935) was born two years after his own birth. It was a strongly Christian atmosphere as might be expected to be found in a Lutheran pastor's home. The household was a little unusual as Pastor Nietzsche's mother and two sisters lived with them, somewhat overshadowing the role of the youthful old Frau Pastor. The most important influence was that of Pastor Nietzsche himself. The father seemed to have an unusual relationship with his young son, allowing him to stay in his study while he was working and often playing the piano in his presence, which enthralled the boy who was still in a toddler stage. There is general agreement that father and son had a special relationship which endured in Nietzsche's mind up until the end of his productive life. All the more tragic was the effect of the death of Pastor Nietzsche when his son was not yet five years old. The loss of his father created a certain disposition to melancholia in Nietzsche's psyche that was to become more prominent in later years.

After the father's death, the family had to leave the parsonage to make room for a newly appointed pastor. Largely on the initiative of the grandmother, the family moved to Naumburg, a larger town in which *Grossmutter* Nietzsche had many connections. Fritz attended the local public school where he encountered a whole new circle of acquaintances. It appears that from the beginning, young Nietzsche was perceived as a different type of personality than the run of the mill Naumburg student. He was precocious in his interests, reserved in his demeanor, and generally isolated from the other boys. Later, when he attended *Gymnasium* in Naumburg, he developed a small group of close friends who tended to look up to him as a superior personality.[1] Some of this information may be slanted as it derives from the recollection of friends long after the time period when Nietzsche had already become famous. However, it tallies with other evidence of Nietzsche's precocity as a child.

There is no question that young Nietzsche was highly gifted in several areas. His musical interests developed early, he was an accomplished piano player by his teens and an ardent devotee of classical German music. At fourteen years of age, he wrote an essay *On Music* embodying his ideas about the significance of music for the human spirit. He composed various pieces for piano, often dedicated to specific individuals. No doubt this dedication to music stemmed in large part from his early experiences of his father at the piano.

Besides music, he exhibited an early attraction to literature. Books exerted a compelling attraction upon him. He loved to visit his grandfather Oehler's parsonage where there was a library in which he could browse. "Best of all was when I could hang about in Grandfather's study room and my greatest pleasure was to browse through the old books and magazines."[2] He composed many poems which demonstrate a remarkable intellectuality for a boy in his early teens. Not only did he compose poems, but he wrote down prose critiques of his own poetry! In the summer of 1858, when not yet fourteen years, he wrote a draft titled *Out of My Life*, presumably inspired by the well-known autobiographical work of Goethe. All in all, the creative energy and talent of the young teenager was a clear harbinger of the things to come.

Given Nietzsche's family heritage, there was an unspoken expectation that he too would become a pastor. His personality and interests gave every indication that this would be the right path for him to follow. A cursory reading of his youthful writings indicate that he was a seriously spiritual young man. Yet he also felt that he had a vocation for a musical career. In this phase of his life, there was a conflict between theology and music for his future career choice. Whichever he chose, however, Nietzsche seemed destined to become an exceptional adult personality.

The shadows that darkened his life at this time were vision problems and severe headaches. Already at four years of age on the recommendation of his grandmother, Nietzsche was taken to see Dr. Ernst Schillbach, professor of ophthalmology at the University of Jena. Schillbach diagnosed myopia of different grades in either eye and anisocoria (unequal diameter of the pupils).[3] Apparently Nietzsche inherited his myopia from his father and the anisocoria from the mother who demonstrated similar pupillary inequalities. This latter condition is ordinarily without clinical significance when existing as an inborn trait but it became quite significant for Nietzsche because it was part of the evidence later used to support a diagnosis of general paresis—syphilitic disease of the brain.

The eyestrain and headaches gradually increased as Nietzsche grew older. Glasses were prescribed by Dr. Schillbach but apparently the symptoms were not relieved. They became significantly worse when in 1858 Nietzsche enrolled in the rigorous boarding school for classical studies at Pforta. All this makes clear that Nietzsche's headaches and ocular problems significantly antedated any possible contraction of a syphilitic infection.

In 1858, Nietzsche's exceptional abilities were recognized by the offer of a full scholarship to the famous classical school at Pforta which many eminent German scholars and writers had attended. It was a boarding school analogous to the elite private preparatory schools of England. Teaching was heavily oriented to classical and humanistic studies. Hayman succinctly summarizes the atmosphere of Pforta:

Built in the twelfth century as a Cistercian abbey, with walls twelve feet high and two and a half feet thick, it was isolated in a valley about four miles from Naumburg. For a Lutheran establishment, the educational system was oddly close to that of the Jesuits. Cloistered behind thick walls, the boys were cut off from the contemporary world. They saw no newspapers and the education was calculated to steep their minds in the classical past. They had six hours of Greek every week throughout their six years at school, eleven hours of Latin weekly during the first three years and ten during their last three. . . . What was peculiarly Prussian about the school was the emphasis on efficiency and the blend of militarism with classicism. . . . Pforta was geared to the same paradoxical combination of asceticism and classicism that had characterized Frederick the Great's court: Voltaire described it as "Sparta in the morning and Athens in the afternoon."[4]

It was here that Nietzsche spent six years from the ages of fourteen to twenty. He felt it to be the most formative period of his life. He learned discipline and perseverance in addition to the intimate knowledge of classical antiquity which marked his cultural orientation throughout the rest of his productive years. But his health paid a price. The poor lighting in the Spartan rooms was terrible for his eyes. The Pforta health records reveal a continuous series of problems.[5] Rheumatism, colds, and headaches were the most frequent entries. It must be remembered that these were only the entries in the health log; given the Spartan atmosphere, it is probable that most of Nietzsche's problems went unrecorded. In the summer of 1856 when he was twelve years old, he had to prolong his summer vacation because of headaches. The school physician was aware of Nietzsche's father's early death and implied in one notation that he was concerned about a similar problem existing in young Nietzsche.

Nietzsche missed a considerable number of classes because of his problems, especially the headaches. These latter caused him to spend many days in the poorly equipped infirmary. Headaches were treated by Dr. Zimmerman, the school physician, with leeches or cupping to draw blood from the affected area. On occasion, Spanish flies (blister beetles attached to the skin to create counter-irritation) were attached behind each ear. One can imagine how these archaic medical practices might have affected the sensitive young patient. Nietzsche's letters to his mother are heart-wrenching, describing continuous headaches preventing him from working or sleeping. The slightest movement of his head would cause pain. At times it was necessary for Nietzsche to return home to Naumburg where he could rest and recover.

It is notable that at this time Nietzsche exhibited painful "rheumatic attacks." They seemed to involve his whole body and were worse when sitting or standing, requiring him to remain in bed. Pains in the neck and throat were part of the "rheumatic" picture. Dr. Zimmerman also treated "rheumatism" with Spanish flies. It is worth noting at this point that similar symptoms occurring in 1865, one year after leaving Pforta, were retrospectively diagnosed by later commentators as stemming from early meningitis consequent to a syphilitic infection.

In spite of his physical problems, Nietzsche was able to maintain his scholastic status, a sign of his superior intelligence and of his ambitious nature. He graduated with outstanding grades with the exception of mathematics which was always a problem for him. His instructor in Latin regarded him as the most gifted student he had ever taught at Pforta. A similar view was expressed years later by Ritschl, his mentor of philology at Leipzig. Unfortunately for Nietzsche, his afflictions were to return in later years with increased force when it was not possible for him to return, either physically or psychologically, to his family home in Naumburg.

3

University Student

After six grueling years at Pforta, Nietzsche felt the desire to experience life directly instead of through the prism of books. In 1864, he and his Pforta schoolmate Paul Deussen undertook a holiday trip to the Rhineland where Deussen's family lived. It was Nietzsche's first excursion away from the Saxony-Thuringia regions of Prussia where he had grown up and attended school. The Rhineland was a more cosmopolitan area of the still piecemeal German collection of petty states. Part of the time, they stayed in Deussen's family home near Coblentz. Like Nietzsche, Deussen was a pastor's son, increasing the experiences they had in common.

Paul Deussen is an invaluable source of information about Nietzsche during his student days. He was an objective yet insightful observer of the young Nietzsche. Later, there was a falling-out between them, principally due to Nietzsche's supersensitive nature. Deussen went on to become professor of philosophy at the University of Kiel and one of Germany's foremost Sanskrit scholars. His book *The Philosophy of the Upanishads* is a classic which has been translated into many languages. It was Deussen who provided the famous story of Nietzsche in a brothel in Cologne to be described later.

At this time in his life, Nietzsche was still vacillating between career choices. His first love was music but he had not been notably successful in attracting attention to his compositions while a life as a performing musician was not at all congruent with his personality. His mother had her heart set on his following in his father's footsteps so, after considerable indecision, he decided to enroll as a theology student at the University of Bonn. Bonn appealed to him because Paul Deussen had enrolled there as well and also because of the strength of its philology department. Nietzsche was drawn to philology because it embodied a "scientific" aspect to classical studies that satisfied the scholarly side of his personality. He thought he could concentrate on the philological study of the Greek Gospels as part of his theological program at Bonn. At Pforta, classical philology was regarded as a science. Today, it would be categorized as the study of classical languages (Greek and Latin) and be included in the humanities division of most universities.

As part of his feeling that he should have a broader experience of life, Nietzsche joined Franconia, one of the student fraternities or *Burschenschaften*, a notorious university phenomenon in the mid-nineteenth century, oriented to a more liberal and united Germany. Hayman suggests that these fraternities provided the background for the *Hitler Jugend* movement of the Third Reich.[1] Of the 29 Franconians at Bonn, 27 were from Pforta. They drank, caroused, and paraded. Dueling was part of the ethos and Nietzsche acquired a dueling scar on the bridge of his nose. The duel was instigated by Nietzsche by means of a polite request made of a casual acquaintance. The details of the incident are known through Deussen and are described in detail by Hayman.

It is clear from Nietzsche's own remembrances and those of other observers that he never was a full-fledged participant in the boisterous fraternity life. He had no capacity to let off steam and apparently no inclination toward sexual experience. As befit a Pforta graduate, Deussen's comment was *"mulierem nunquam attigit"*—he never touched a woman. Nietzsche could not divest himself of his deeply rooted seriousness and orientation to abstract thought. Another student acquaintance said of him, "he was no gay blade (*lustiger Student*) and never showed the need to have a fling."[2]

It was during this period that Deussen recounts the notorious brothel episode as Nietzsche described it to him. Bonn students were accustomed to visit houses of ill repute in Cologne, some distance downstream on the Rhine. One day, Nietzsche was alone in Cologne and, according to Deussen, asked a porter to guide him to some interesting sights (*Sehenswürdigkeiten*). The porter guided him to a brothel where he suddenly found himself surrounded by a half dozen scantily clad creatures who looked at him expectantly. For a moment he was speechless and paralyzed. Then he caught sight of a piano as the single spiritual thing in the room and instinctively sat down at it to play a chord. This released him from his paralysis and he fled the house to freedom.[3] Thomas Mann later used this episode in his fictional account of a Nietzsche-like personality in *Dr. Faustus*.

One may wonder if the visit really was accidental as told by Deussen. But there is no reason to doubt the events occurred as he described. Nietzsche may have gotten cold feet when confronted with the reality of a sexual encounter at that time. However, it seems clear from recent evidence that Nietzsche had had sexual liaisons and had acquired gonorrhea (*Der Tripper*, the clap) during his student days.[4] He probably regarded it as no more than a minor inconvenience. No mention was ever made of syphilis by Nietzsche. The assumption that he contracted syphilis rests on the assumption that because he developed general paresis, he must have acquired this disease at some earlier time in his life. But Nietzsche, who was very forthcoming to his friends and doctors about every aspect of his life including graphic descriptions of all his illnesses, never mentioned anything in either his letters or his notebooks about a diagnosis of or treatment for syphilis.

Generally, Nietzsche was in much better health in Bonn as compared to his Pforta years. Little is said about headaches or eye problems. However, toward the end of his residence in Bonn, there occurred a repeat of the "rheumatism" which he had suffered in Pforta. Pain occurred in his arms, neck, back, and finally culminated in severe headaches. These lasted for some weeks forcing him to remain in bed. It is not clear whether these were an unusual feature of his tendency to migraine or some other condition, perhaps a flu-like disorder. Nietzsche himself tried to recover through limiting his exposure to excitation and taking recourse to dietary regimes. Janz suggests that Nietzsche always exhibited bodily symptoms when he was at a crossroads in his life, in this case, the significant impending move from Bonn to Leipzig.[5]

Nietzsche became increasingly ambivalent about his theological studies in Bonn, especially because it was an expensive place to live, causing him recurrent financial worries. Finally, he made a bold decision to change his venue to Leipzig in order to concentrate solely on philological studies. The fact that his major professor of philology at Bonn, Ritschl, was moving to Leipzig confirmed him in his decision. His mother was outraged and brought to tears by his decision to leave theology but Nietzsche stuck to his decision. In October 1865, he transferred to Leipzig.

The two years Nietzsche spent as a graduate student in Leipzig were perhaps the most healthy and happy years for him. He was a brilliant student, impressing Ritschl greatly with his originality and maturity. His interests in philosophy were greatly stimulated by his discovery of Schopenhauer while browsing through a Leipzig bookstore. The latter's forceful style and freedom of expression had a profound effect on him, at least as much as did Schopenhauer's ideas themselves. The impact of Schopenhauer can be seen in Nietzsche's uninhibited and freewheeling style of expression.

Cholera broke out in Naumburg while Nietzsche was home on vacation causing him and his mother to flee to a neighboring town. His sister told the story that Nietzsche thought he was infected on two different occasions by cholera and cured himself through drinking large quantities of hot water. Memory of these two "infections" may have been in his mind over twenty years later when totally psychotic in a Basel institution, he claimed to have infected himself twice. The Basel psychiatrists thought he meant syphilis. Hildebrandt provides a detailed discussion of this episode.[6] A more likely possibility, deriving from the *Tripper* information mentioned above and not available to Hildebrandt, was that Nietzsche was referring to treatment for gonorrhea.

The Leipzig period is also responsible for another one of those strange tales which seem to attach themselves to the Nietzsche chronicles. Wilhelm Lange-Eichbaum was a Berlin psychiatrist who in 1931 had published an article in a medical journal titled *Nietzsche as a Psychiatric Problem*. As a result of this publication, he received a communication from a "prominent" Berlin neurologist (unnamed) who said that Nietzsche had contracted syphilis in a Leipzig bordello for which he had been treated by two Leipzig physicians (unnamed). Lange-Eichbaum goes on to provide the following additional "data." Möbius who had lived in Leipzig at that time had possessed letters from these physicians (never mentioned by Möbius in his monograph). The letters were later destroyed. A well-known pathographic writer (unnamed) wrote to a German medical weekly (unreferenced) that he—the unnamed pathographic writer—had the story confirmed by Möbius' brother and by the son of one of the physicians (both unnamed). All this was described in a monograph Lange-Eichbaum published fifteen years later, afterwards reviewed by Volz who noted the many uncertainties of the account.[7,8]

Lange-Eichbaum may be forgiven for having published this story in 1946. His homeland had just emerged from the long nightmare of 1933–1945. Concealment and vagueness were probably a part of German life during this period. However, it is not appropriate to lend credence to such stories which appropriately fall into the category of gossip. Why are none of these people named? Who knows what the motives may be for such stories? Was the Leipzig bordello confused with the Cologne bordello? Nietzsche may have been treated by doctors in Leipzig, but for what reason? Could he have feared syphilis and sought out prophylactic treatment? Syphilophobia was widespread in Europe at the time and had affected none other than Schopenhauer who had more reason for concern. One can conjecture at length on the subject but there is no reliable information and the tale does not belong in serious discussions of Nietzsche's medical history.

As a citizen of Prussia, Nietzsche had an obligation for military service. In September 1867 he passed the medical examination by using weak glasses to fake the severity of his myopia. He enlisted in an artillery regiment stationed in Naumburg so that he could live at home with his family. Part of the training involved horseback riding at which Nietzsche excelled. However, perhaps because of his myopia, he misjudged mounting his horse and threw himself against the saddle pommel. A severe chest injury ensued which suppurated and spread to the underlying sternum. Five months of treatment of abscesses and bone infection were required. Janz suggests this illness initiated Nietzsche's preoccupation with the effect of illness on his life and thought.

Nietzsche returned to Leipzig after his year of military service. There he met Richard Wagner who was the second person—Schopenhauer was the first—to have a profound impact on him. Wagner seemed to embody all the features that he found missing in the stodgy milieu of university life; Wagner was creative, intense, philosophically-minded, and engaged in real life activities. Nietzsche was dazzled by the impact of his personality and later was to become an enthusiastic participant in the activities of the Wagnerian circle.

Ritschl continued to be impressed by Nietzsche, recommending him for the professorship in philology at the University of Basel which had recently become vacant. It was an unusual recommendation since Nietzsche was only 24 years old and had not yet received his doctorate. However Ritschl, who was otherwise an experienced academician and cautious personality, in this case exhibited no reservations. He wrote to the Basel search committee that he had never in his 39-year career had a student as brilliant as Nietzsche. He would be capable of doing "whatever he wished." This was an unconsciously prophetic statement of Ritschl's who did not suspect what Nietzsche ultimately would wish to do. The appointment was offered to Nietzsche in early February 1869. He departed Leipzig for Basel in April 1869.

Nietzsche was asked by his new Swiss employers whether he would apply for Swiss citizenship. It was implied that this would be desirable for his new post. This step required him to give up his Prussian citizenship which he soon formally renounced. The Swiss citizenship, however, would not be forthcoming for an extended period of time because of residency requirements. Thus Nietzsche became a "stateless" person, a situation which came to have much meaning for him. He became and remained in his heart a "European."

The appointment represented a radical change in Nietzsche's circumstances because he suddenly vaulted from insecure student status to a full tenured professorship. It was not a step he took lightly and, at least to his friends and relatives, exhibited many hesitations about entering into his new duties. He knew he would be giving up his freedom for creative work in music and philosophy. To his mother and sister who were overjoyed by his sudden appointment to such a prestigious post, he wrote in February 1869, "What's at the core of this glorious position? Sweat and struggle." In this, as in many other things, Nietzsche had a foreboding of what was to come.

4

Basel Professor

One could make a strong case for an argument that the appointment of Nietzsche as a professor of philology at the age of 24 years was a catastrophe for him. Suddenly he was lifted out of his free life as a private instructor and doctoral student in Leipzig into the demanding tasks of a Swiss university professor. At Basel, he had substantial commitments as a teacher in the *Gymnasium* (high school) as well as his university work. On top of that, he was expected to deliver frequent public lectures. From the beginning, Nietzsche felt himself to be overburdened and distracted from his true mission in life. He believed that he was destined to be more than a "schoolmaster" which was how he designated his professorial work. A feeling of importance in his position as "professor"—the compensation for many overworked people in higher education—never really was a factor in Nietzsche's psychology. On the contrary, he had to struggle against an emotion of contempt toward his surroundings, a sense that he was trapped in a limited bourgeois world oriented only to utilitarian concerns and blind to all higher aspirations. Throughout his career as professor, Nietzsche was always on the lookout for some way to escape from it.

For the first few years of Nietzsche's teaching career, he struggled manfully to fulfill his university commitments and also to look toward his own personal development. During the early Basel years, the most important element in Nietzsche's self-image as a creative person was his relationship with Richard Wagner. He had first met Wagner in Leipzig and had become enthralled with Wagner's style and scope. One of the advantages connected with Nietzsche's relocation to Basel was its relative closeness to *Tribschen*, Wagner's isolated country villa near Lake Lucerne. Soon after his arrival in Basel, and in spite of his heavy teaching load, Nietzsche undertook an uninvited visit to Wagner's villa. The road only went as far as the town of Lucerne; there, one had to take a steamer to a remote village and hike to the villa. It was an audacious act on Nietzsche's part to present himself without an invitation.

Nevertheless, all went well. Cosima von Bülow, Wagner's mistress and later his wife (herself the daughter of Franz Liszt), remembered Nietzsche from Leipzig and was impressed by his professorial title. She permitted access to the "Master." Throughout Nietzsche's long relationship with Wagner and, as later events indicated, his own infatuation with Cosima, she could rarely bring herself to refer to Nietzsche as anything other than "Professor Nietzsche." (Wagner felt otherwise, he often urged Nietzsche to give up his demanding schoolmaster's position.) The visit was a success, Nietzsche and Wagner got on well together and the former became a regular house guest at *Tribschen*, participating in the small social circle of Wagner's admirers. "The isle of the blessed" was how he referred to *Tribschen* during his early years at Basel. But this feeling was soon to change.

The Franco-Prussian War (1870–1871) provided an interlude to Nietzsche's stressful life in Basel. In spite of his relinquishment of Prussian citizenship, Nietzsche still had feelings for his native land. He felt he owed something to Prussia which had provided him with an outstanding education and in which his family still lived. He applied for a leave from his university post in order to volunteer as a medical orderly in the Prussian army. His days as an artillerist were over; he thought he could best serve in caring for the wounded and diseased, an indication perhaps, that his sense of himself as a European had progressed greatly since 1867.

A ten day course in front line medical care was given to all medical orderlies prior to being sent to the war zone. There he learned first hand about medicine and gained the familiarity with medications that he was later to display with respect to his own illnesses. His first major assignment was with the wounded, following the bloody battle of Wörth. He was required to care for six wounded men being returned from the front lines on a hospital train. They were all severely wounded with accompanying dysentery, diphtheria, and gangrene. Nietzsche had difficulty coping with the stark horror of the situation. He himself finally caught diphtheria and dysentery.[1] Some weeks of hospitalization and convalescence were required before he could return to teaching. The possibility is raised by Hildebrandt that Nietzsche might have acquired an extragenital syphilis at that time.[2] The conjecture is impossible to prove or disprove. Generally, extragenital syphilis is regarded as a unusual circumstance.

In October 1870, Nietzsche returned to his professorial duties. His feeling that he was misplaced as a professor of philology had intensified. Many signs gave evidence to his discontent. When in early 1871 the chair of philosophy at Basel became vacant, he proposed to the university governing board that he be appointed to the chair while recommending his friend Erwin Rohde for the post in philology which he would vacate. His proposal was not accepted. An even more radical sign of his disaffection occurred when Cosima wrote to ask whether he could recommend someone to accompany a young prince on a world tour to Italy, Greece, the East, and America. Nietzsche recommended himself (!)—it would be his chance to escape from the chains of the university. Cosima thought it unthinkable that he should give up his chair and he submitted to her judgement.[3] However, it was another piece of evidence that all was not well behind the professorial facade.

Meanwhile, Nietzsche's health was again causing him serious concern. For the first time, he was having stomach problems on top of his other symptoms. Eyestrain, headaches, and vomiting gradually worsened. Minor illnesses such as hemorrhoids and shingles were annoyances. He felt in 1873 that "the machine was breaking down." It was during this time that he began his dabbling with a multitude of treatments for his symptoms, interspersed with consultations with various physicians. Leeches and cupping were again used as in his Pforta days. Diets, hydrotherapies, physical therapies, electrotherapies, all kinds of medications, and home remedies were tried by him at different times. He was a voracious reader of medical and physiological texts. Volz provides a compendium of Nietzsche's involvement with "cures" of every type.[4] In spite of his critical spirit, he seemed to be unduly credulous of every new cure that came to his attention. In the long run, none of them did him any good.

What Nietzsche really desired was to withdraw into an informal private world which he was always trying to construct. There was the constant dream that he could find a small circle of like-minded friends with whom he could pursue his philosophical interests. When he discovered the Alps, he found he could disappear from the world through long walks in the forests, sometimes up to six to eight hours. Later, in *Human, All Too Human, s*. 283, he commented that anyone who does not have two-thirds of the day to himself is a slave, whatever else he may be: statesman, merchant, official, scholar. He was tired of what he felt to be the slavery of professorial life.

Kurt Hildebrandt, chief physician at a psychiatric clinic in Berlin, provided an extensive analysis of Nietzsche's medical problems in the previously cited 1925 monograph *Health and Illness in Nietzsche's Life and Work*. It is still one of the best books on the subject. Hildebrandt advances the thesis that Nietzsche's illnesses prior to his breakdown of 1888 were largely psychosomatic in nature. In Basel, they were a means of his escaping the obligations of work, and later, a means of escaping the pressures to participate in the Wagner idolatry occurring in Bayreuth which Nietzsche had gradually come to loathe. Migraine, from which Nietzsche suffered (a family trait affecting his father and sister), is a classical form of psychosomatic illness. The headaches, vomiting, and prostration are physical symptoms brought on by emotional strains or pressures. Möbius, who was an expert on migraine as well as a sufferer himself, had no doubt that Nietzsche was afflicted with the disorder. Weak vision was certainly also a major contributor to Nietzsche's problems as his profession required a great deal of reading. However in his good periods, Nietzsche was able to function quite well with his limited visual capacities.

Nietzsche's publications during his tenure at Basel were further evidence of his conflicted attitude toward academic life. His first book publication in 1872, *The Birth of Tragedy*, was an intuitive essay dealing with the origins of Greek tragedy. Later, the British classicist, F.M. Cornford was to say of it that it was "a work of profound imaginative insight, which left the scholarship of a generation toiling in the rear."[5] However, at the time, it was seen as a self-indulgent writing exhibiting none of the qualities expected of scholarly work. There were no references, no notes, none of the usual scholarly apparatus expected of a newly appointed university professor. It was attacked publicly and was responsible for Nietzsche's virtual ostracism from contemporary classical philology in the German-speaking world. Philology students stopped coming to his lectures. However, Nietzsche was not dissuaded from his desire to engage in innovative, philosophical writing no matter how unscholarly they might appear to conventional university faculty. His four *Untimely Meditations*, essays on contemporary issues, and his first book of aphorisms, *Human, All Too Human* all appeared while he was teaching at Basel. None of them could do anything for his reputation as a professor because they were personal rather than scholarly expositions.

In 1876, he requested a leave of absence from the university on the grounds of illness. It was granted giving Nietzsche a prolonged time period away from Basel. It was during this period that he discovered Italy, a place where he felt a sense of liberation compared to what he felt to be the heavy atmosphere of the German northlands. A long-standing woman friend, Malwida von Meysenbug, had invited him for a prolonged stay at her villa in Sorrento. He spent the winter of 1876–1877 in Sorrento where he was able to live an idyllic life, discussing philosophy with a few close friends and gradually developing his concepts. By and large, he was healthier during this period although headaches still occurred. Subsequently, he traveled throughout Italy and then back to the Alps during the summer. It was during this period that he met Dr. Otto Eiser, an admirer of his writings, who felt that Nietzsche had not received consistent medical care and suggested he visit Eiser's office in Frankfurt for a thorough evaluation of all of his medical problems. Nietzsche was later to accept this offer.

After his return to Basel in 1877, Nietzsche's condition became much worse. He would become virtually blind at times and headaches incapacitated him after every attempt at lecturing. His sister lived with him for a period of time but she was no real help to him. His letters to friends and family are filled with a feeling of despair about his health. In spite of all these woes, however, he continued to work on *Human, All Too Human* which was published in 1878.

Throughout all the frequent changes of venue, Nietzsche continued to seek medical treatments. One has the feeling of a certain obsessive-compulsive quality to his endless focusing on his illnesses. In a letter to his sister on December 29, 1879, he describes 118 "attacks" for the year not yet over, a revealing confession of preoccupation with counting symptoms. Furthermore, it is clear that Nietzsche was able to proceed with his own personal writing regardless of illness and demands of his profession. All this is not to say that he feigned illness, there can be no doubt that his vision deteriorated and his headaches were so severe that at times he felt himself to be on the edge of death.

In October 1877, he traveled to Frankfurt for an extended consultation with Dr. Otto Eiser, the physician he had met in the Swiss Alps the previous summer. Dr. Eiser subjected him to an extensive evaluation, including an examination by an ophthalmologist colleague, Dr. Gustav Kruger. A written report was provided by Dr. Eiser which is given in full by Volz.[6] The essence of the report indicated that Nietzsche had bilateral inflammation of the inner layers of the eyes, *chorioretinitis centralis*. This disorder was thought to be responsible, at least in part, for Nietzsche's headaches. Heroic treatment interventions were to be avoided. The most important thing was "absolute avoidance of reading and writing for a number of years (!) with avoidance of the use of concave glasses (which had been prescribed for Nietzsche's myopia). Blue sunglasses were recommended to avoid light stimulation. Cold water baths and other "toughening" exercises were to be avoided. In general, all types of excessive stimulation were prohibited, including strong coffee, tea, and heavy wine.

Recently, supplemental information has come to light regarding this consultation.[7] Dr. Eiser took the ethically dubious step of providing specifics of the consultation to Richard Wagner who also knew Eiser and maintained a strong interest in Nietzsche's health. Today such a step would be considered an absolute breach of medical confidentiality. Wagner had suspected *Onanie*—masturbation—to be at the root of Nietzsche's problems but Eiser informed Wagner that there was no evidence such was the case. In fact, Nietzsche, according to Eiser, had admitted engaging in sexual relations on several occasions on the advice of a physician. Additionally, he admitted to having been infected with gonorrhea—*Tripper*—on two occasions during his student days. He specifically denied ever having contracted syphilis which Eiser accepted as a valid statement. (So much for the views of Nietzsche's friends that he had never touched a woman.) Further, Eiser makes the relevant point that most people affected by Nietzsche's type of eye problems do not have such severe headaches so that some other factor must be present. This of course would be migraine which Eiser does not mention. Additionally, Dr. Kruger's prohibition of concave lenses is an implied acknowledgment that overcorrection or unequal correction of Nietzsche's myopia may have been a contributory factor to his eyestrain and headaches.

After receiving this report, Nietzsche applied for an additional six month leave of absence from his *Gymnasium* responsibilities. However, he continued to teach intermittently at the university. A last ophthalmological consultation was obtained with the noted Dr. Alfred Graefe in Halle. Graefe was very pessimistic about preservation of Nietzsche's eyesight in his university circumstances. Thereupon, in July 1879, he finally submitted a complete resignation from his post at the University of Basel. It was accepted and he was awarded a pension that was about two thirds of his salary as an active professor.

During Nietzsche's early Basel years, he composed a manuscript titled *Philosophy in the Tragic Age of the Greeks*. It stems from the same period as *The Birth of Tragedy* but was never published during Nietzsche's lifetime. One of the notebook entries during this period seems not to have been included in the manuscript. It is a statement of an imaginary last philosopher, Oedipus, named after the Sophoclean tragic hero. Like virtually all of Nietzsche's depictions, it is essentially a picture of himself—a self which was presumably not noticed by most of his Basel colleagues. The role of Oedipus in the passage is obscure but the meaning of the passage is chillingly clear. It is an anticipation of Nietzsche's own total alienation from his society.

Oedipus
Conversations of the Last Philosopher with Himself
A Fragment from the Annals of Posterity

The last philosopher I call myself since I am the last human being. No one speaks with me except myself and my voice sounds to me as one dying. With you, beloved voice, with you, my last breath of memory of all human joy, let me reminisce for but an hour, escaping solitude and deluding myself into love and friendship since my heart resists believing that love is dead; it cannot bear the horror of unbroken solitude, it forces me to speak as if I were two.

Do I still hear you, my voice? You whisper while you curse? Shall not your curse burst the entrails of this world? But the world lives on; glowing coldly, its merciless stars stare at me; it lives on, blind and deaf as always, and only one thing dies, the human being.

And yet! I hear you yet, beloved voice! There dies yet another in this world besides myself, the last human being; there dies the last sorrower with me in protracted misery. Woe! Woe! Beside me mourns Oedipus, the last woebegone man.[8]

5

Homeless Philosopher

Following his resignation from the University of Basel, Nietzsche went through a period of prolonged indecision as to his next steps. His meager furniture and book collection were sold by his sister Elisabeth after his departure from Basel. He spent some weeks in St. Moritz where he met Elisabeth who thought he looked much better compared to his last winter in Basel when Nietzsche thought himself to be near death. Nietzsche knew of an empty tower on an abandoned part of the city wall near his mother's house in Naumburg. There was a small garden attached to it. He was able to arrange for its rental and in September 1879 he moved into the area. He began writing while cultivating the garden in his free time.

From the beginning, it was not a happy arrangement. He injured his back working in the garden. The headaches recurred with increased frequency so even before the end of 1879 he calculated that he had 118 days of headaches during the year. He felt that the cold, snowy weather of Naumburg was terrible for him. He wrote his friend Malwida von Meysenbug on January 14, 1880:

Although writing for me belongs to forbidden fruit, yet, since I love and honor you as an elder sister, you shall have one more letter from me—

it may well be the last. Since the fearful and unrelenting torture of my life causes me to yearn for the end, and there are signs that an impending stroke is close enough to hope for it.

In a similar tone, Nietzsche wrote to Dr. Eiser in early January 1880:

My existence is a *fearful* burden: I would have long thrown it over if I had not been making the most instructive tests and experiments in the spiritual-moral area in exactly this condition of suffering and of enduring almost total deprivation—this pleasure in knowledge brings me to heights in which I am victorious over all tortures and all hopelessness. In general, I am happier than I have ever been and yet! Constant pain, a feeling of semi-paralysis something like sea-sickness in which speaking is difficult for me alternating with raging attacks (the last one caused me vomiting for three days and nights, I longed for death). Not to be able to read! Rarely able to write! No intercourse with people! Unable to listen to music! To be alone, to walk alone, a diet of milk, eggs and mountain air. Unable to help myself, nothing is useful to me. The cold hurts me. I am going south sometime during the next few weeks to begin a walking-existence. My *consolation* is in my thoughts and perspectives. I scribble while walking on a sheet of paper, I write nothing at my desk, a friend deciphers my scribbling. [Peter Gast, who wrote the first draft of many of his manuscripts]

Perhaps more relevant to this situation is a letter he later wrote on March 6, 1883, to Overbeck, his closest Basel friend:

Breaking away from my relatives was the beginning of really doing something for myself; oh, if you knew what I have had to overcome in my life since my birth! I do not like my mother, and listening to my sister's voice makes me miserable; I have always been sick when I was together with them.

Finally, Nietzsche decided to leave Naumburg for good. He made arrangements to meet his young friend and admirer Peter Gast (a.k.a. Heinrich Köselitz) in Italy with Venice to be their final destination. The departure from his family and Germany was the last step in Nietzsche's separation from his old life. The Basel professorship had been given up, now he was to become an expatriate in foreign lands, far from family and friends. He had freed himself from the burdens of university teaching and the strains of family connections; now he was to encounter a new problem, that of the lonely émigré. Aside from his physical complaints, loneliness was the main thing he complained of in his letters. It was to be expected that his loneliness would give way to depression. Jacob Burckhardt already noticed this tendency in Nietzsche early during the Basel years but the problem greatly intensified as a consequence of his isolation in the non-German speaking areas to which he had fled. Nietzsche did not have a flair for speaking other languages and although he spent ten years largely in France and Italy, his command of spoken French was poor and of Italian even poorer.

Janz has labeled the period 1879–1889 of Nietzsche's life as ten years as a free philosopher but it can also be regarded as ten years of homelessness. There was no fixed abode during this period, no place he could call his own; there was only the constant succession of usually dreary *pensions de famille* in the French or Italian Rivieras or summer resorts in the Swiss Alps where Nietzsche felt contempt for the German tourists who frequented them. A rough calculation reveals that there were 46 changes of geographical locale during these ten years but this does not count all the changes of residence within specific locales. Nietzsche himself noted that during seven winters in Genoa and Nice, he had rented 21 rooms. His modest library, notes and manuscripts followed via all kinds of shipping arrangements. His visual disability approached near total blindness on occasion. It is really quite amazing that he was able to accomplish any writing at all. Yet he authored eleven books during this period, eight of which he saw through to final publication; the other three appeared posthumously. Along with his formal writing, he engaged in an enormous correspondence that composes an important part of the Nietzsche literary corpus. It is hard to think of any other writer who had to overcome so many obstacles during his main creative period. No doubt this is why Nietzsche set such store on the concept of *Selbstüberwindung*—self-overcoming—as a necessary feature of personal development.

It is not easy to understand exactly why Nietzsche had such a compulsion to move about. It must have been extraordinarily difficult for him to constantly arrange for new lodgings, become familiar with new neighborhoods, organize transportation of his possessions—all with his poor vision and, with the exception of his Swiss residences, limited skills with the local languages. He dwells greatly on climate as the reason for many of his changes. Too much sun was bad for his eyes, too much cold produced blue fingers and exacerbated his headaches, too much humidity was bad for his digestion. One has trouble imagining that a person of such superior intelligence as Nietzsche could have set such store on climatic conditions. He seemed to be a person who could not sit still, much of his day when he was not writing was spent walking, often up to six to eight hours at a time in spite of his poor vision. There was a demon within Nietzsche that gave him no rest.

While he continued to have frequent headaches with vomiting and complained of his bad vision, his health was by and large better than it had been in Basel. He felt that he had passed a turning point during the illnesses of 1879–1880 when he had felt on the verge of death. He no longer visited doctors as he had so frequently done during the Basel years, partly, no doubt, because of his more restricted financial situation, but also because he had given up expecting much from the medical profession. Photographs and descriptions of him during this period indicate that he had stopped wearing glasses. He felt he had taken charge of his own health, and, if not able to cure himself, at least he was able to keep his illnesses at bay. He wrote in *Ecce Homo* (Why I Am So Wise, *s*.2):

The energy for absolute solitude and release from customary relationships, my insistence on not allowing myself to be cared for, to be served, to be doctored—that revealed an absolute certainty of instinct about what was necessary at that time. I took myself in hand, I made myself healthy again; the prerequisite for this—every physiologist would agree—*is that a person be fundamentally healthy.*

Embedded in Nietzsche's overall feeling of misery is described what appears to be a severe attack of migraine. Loneliness, depression, visual loss, and migraine were the witches' brew that tortured him during this time. Only the activities of his mind gave him relief.

The image that emerges of Nietzsche during his ten years as a homeless philosopher greatly varies according to the sources. There are Nietzsche's own letters that give different pictures to different people and there are the descriptions of Nietzsche given by his friends. His letters to Franz Overbeck, the loyal friend of his Basel days who handled his modest pension, are invariably gloomy and depressed except for the last few months of 1888 when he had entered into his euphoric stage. He sent at least two hundred letters to Overbeck during the period 1880–1888. Poor Overbeck must have dreaded receiving letters with the familiar tight handwriting on the envelope. It surely accounted for Overbeck's consistently pessimistic view of Nietzsche's prospects, even before his breakdown. The letter of March 22, 1883, from Genoa is characteristic:

My dear friend, I think you haven't written to me in a long time. However, perhaps I deceive myself, the days are so long, I no longer know what I will do with each day: I've lost interest in everything. Deep down, an unmovable black melancholy. Also weariness. Most of the time in bed; it's the most sensible thing for me. I have become quite thin which is surprising; I have a good *trattoria* now and would like to build myself up again. But the worst is: I don't see any more *why* I should live even another half a year, everything is boring, painful, degoutant. I've suffered and sacrificed too much and have a sense of the imperfection, the mistakes and the mishaps of my entire spiritual past life which is beyond all understanding. There is nothing worthwhile to do anymore; I can't create anything any longer. Why try at all!

This after completion of *Thus Spoke Zarathustra*. It was letters such as these that led Overbeck to anticipate a mental breakdown in his friend.

Nietzsche's letters to his family were not dissimilar from those to Overbeck, although to his mother and sister he could be a little more cheerful. But there were other sides to Nietzsche's personality. He could be very serious without a trace of self-pity and even charming on occasion. He shared pension lodgings in Nice during December 1883 with a Viennese Jewish physician, Dr. Joseph Paneth, to whom he felt a certain affinity. They had several serious discussions, unusual for Nietzsche with respect to his fellow lodgers. Paneth later wrote that Nietzsche told him "without the slightest affectation or self-consciousness that he always felt that a task had been assigned to him and now he wanted, as far as his eyes would permit, to work it through...I was amazed that there was nothing effusive or contrived in his demeanor."[1]

Paneth later communicated his experiences with Nietzsche to Sigmund Freud to whose circle he belonged until his own premature death from tuberculosis in 1890.

But an even more uplifting account of Nietzsche was provided by a 29-year-old doctoral student named Resa von Schirnhofer who spent much of her Easter vacation in 1884 with Nietzsche. They corresponded thereafter for several years. There does not seem to be any evidence of a physical or romantic relationship between them. She later described her experiences with Nietzsche at some length:

On first meeting Nietzsche, I felt a certain embarrassment. However, his friendly but dignified manner, his serious professorial appearance, our common motherly friend [Malvida von Meysenbug], who was invisibly present to facilitate matters, soon put me at ease. During the 10 days of my residence on the delightful Côte d'Azure, Nietzsche devoted much of his valuable time to me. He took me to his favorite pathways, we took walks, little outings, enjoyed the magic pleasures of nature and of the climate, he brought me books to look over, others from which I read aloud to him on occasion and however great the distance was between the thinker and writer from the young student, it did not affect the simple human relationship. So uninhibited as a thinker, Nietzsche as a man was exquisitely sensitive, gentle and exceptionally courteous in his attitude and manners toward the female sex. . . . There was nothing in his nature which disturbed me in any way.[2]

No doubt Nietzsche, who was always looking for potential young disciples, put on a performance for Resa. Nevertheless, his relationship with her and other people who interested him reveals that he was not always on the verge of suicide.

Insomnia was a recurrent problem for Nietzsche. He took to using chloral hydrate, a popular sedative at that time, to help him sleep. On February 1, 1883, he wrote to Overbeck that he was no longer able to sleep without the aid of this medication. It is not clear exactly how much and how regularly Nietzsche took chloral hydrate; although, in the same letter, he stated that he took 50 grams over a two-month period. This does not calculate out to a high daily dose if Nietzsche did not take several doses at once. Chloral hydrate is a relatively safe agent without strong addiction properties. Dr. Wille, however, during Nietzsche's institutionalization in Basel, expressed the view that chloral and other medications had affected his mind for a long time.[3] His sister Elisabeth always maintained that use of chloral was the principal reason for his breakdown and Peter Gast was of a similar opinion. The possibility cannot be entirely excluded that it was at least a contributory factor.

Gast brought Nietzsche a typewriter in 1882 but apparently he could never take to its use. Unless he was absolutely incapacitated by illness, he went for frequent walks, several hours at a time. Cold weather bothered him, his fingers would turn blue when he wrote in the winter. Bright light always irritated his eyes; one of the attractions of Turin was that the trees and buildings everywhere protected him from the direct rays of the sun. He drank no wine, beer, spirits, or coffee. Stefan Zweig gives an imaginative account of his life during these years, freely drawing on his own capacity for dramatization, but probably containing far more truth than fiction:

Portrait of the man: A meager dining-room of a six-franc pension in an Alpine hotel or on the Ligurian coast. Mediocre guests, usually elderly women in "small talk." The bell rings three times for dinner. Across the threshold steps a slightly bowed, uncertain figure: as if emerging from a cave, the "six-seventh blind" person always gropes his way into an unfamiliar area. Dark carefully brushed clothes, the face also dark with bushy, brown, wavy hair. The eyes dark as well behind thick round spectacles. Softly, even shyly, he enters, an unusual quietness to his demeanor. One senses a person who lives in the shadows, beyond the society of conversation, for whom all loudness and noise is feared with an almost neurasthenic anxiety: Courteously, with exaggerated manners, he would greet the guests, courteously, with pleasant indifference, the others greeted the German professor. Cautiously, the myopic person drew himself up to the table, cautiously, the dyspeptic person tests every dish: whether the tea was too strong, the food overly spiced, every dietary error would ruin his shaky nerves for days on end. No wine, no beer, no alcohol, no coffee served at his place at the table, no cigar or cigarette after dinner, nothing which cheers, refreshes or relaxes; only the meagre meal and some small, superficial conversation in a soft tone with a chance meal partner (as one speaks who has been unaccustomed to conversation for years and fears to be asked too much).

And again up to the narrow, meager, sparse and coldly furnished *Chambre garnie*, the table heaped up with countless sheets, notes, writings and corrections, no flowers, no ornaments, hardly a book and seldom a letter. Back in a corner, a heavy, clumsy, wooden trunk, his only possession and a second well-worn suit. Otherwise, only books and manu-scripts; on a tray numerous flasks, bottles and tinctures against the headaches which often make him groggy for hours, against stomach cramps, against the retching, against constipation and above all, the fear-ful agents against insomnia, chloral and veronal. A horrible arsenal of drugs and poisons, and yet the only help in this empty silence of a strange room, in which he had no rest except in short, artificially-induced sleep. Wrapped in an overcoat with a muffler around his neck (because the miserable stove merely smoked and didn't heat), with freezing fin-gers, the double lenses pressed close to the paper, the hurrying hand wrote words for hours on end which his clouded eyes could hardly de-cipher himself. He sat for hours in this way, writing, until his eyes burned and teared: it was a rare good fortune when a compassionate person would take dictation from him for an hour or two. In good weather, the solitary figure would go out, always alone, always with his thoughts: never a greeting on the way, never a companion, never a meet-ing. In gray weather which he hated, in rain or snow which hurt his eyes, he had to remain in the prison of his room: he never went to the room of someone else. Only evenings, a couple of cookies, a glass of thin tea, and then again the long, continuous solitude with only his thoughts. He stayed awake for hours by the flickering, smoking lamp, without being able to relax his overstimulated nerves. Then he would reach for the chloral, for any kind of sedative, and finally the sleep which comes easily to other men, less obsessed with ideas and not pursued by de-mons, is forced upon him.

Many times he remains in bed all day. Retching and cramps to the point of unconsciousness, gnawing pains in the temples, almost complete blindness. No one would come to him, no one with a kind hand to place a compress on his forehead, no one to read to him, to chat with him, to laugh with him.

This *Chambre garnie* was the same everywhere. The name of the city changed often, Turin, Venice, Nice, Marienbad, but the *Chambre garnie* was always the same, always the unfamiliar, rented room with old, cold, used furniture, the writing-table, the painful bed and the endless soli-tude.[4]

The picture may be exaggerated. It is the privilege of literary per-sonalities such as Stefan Zweig. However, even if it is only half true, it portrays a grim picture of the conditions under which Nietzsche produced his unique masterpieces.

Shortly after Nietzsche's death, there began to emerge the so-called "pathographic" literature. These were articles, usually of medical origin, in which the authors sought to find evidence in Nietzsche's writings of the effects of syphilis. They began with the publication of a monograph on Nietzsche by Paul Möbius to be discussed in Chapter 10. Möbius believed that all of Nietzsche's works written after 1880 showed the effect of general paresis. The most extensive discussion of this subject was provided by Wilhelm Lange-Eichbaum, a German psychiatrist whose most famous work titled *Genius, Insanity and Fame* was published in 1942. The pathographic writers did not necessarily believe that Nietzsche's work was adversely affected by his paralysis; on the contrary, it was thought by some that the spirochetal disease in the frontal lobe of the brain produced a "disinhibition" which allowed free flow to Nietzsche's innate genius. This was the view of the discussants at the Vienna Psychoanalytic Society meetings in the first decade of the twentieth century.[5] Lange-Eichbaum believed that "the intellectual and philosophical development of the young Nietzsche was significantly fostered and deepened through the agonies of his syphilis and their spiritual effects."[6]

Today, the effort to relate Nietzsche's specific thoughts to a presumed paretic condition is no longer attempted. Yet the opinion generally still exists that his later writings, particularly those of 1888, have been affected by his illness. It is thought that by physiologically releasing inhibitions, the disease acted to exaggerate his pronouncements and to heighten his grandiosity. Some writers have exhibited their own disinhibition by elaborating metaphors such as "the snakes writhe in his consciousness like the spirochaetes curling around his brain tissue" or "as the brain loses mass, the result of tertiary syphilis, the human consciousness seems to effervesce in megalomania."[7] Others are more restrained yet feel that the presence of the paresis with its necessary effects on the personality has been conclusively demonstrated.[8]

Early in the decade of the eighties, Nietzsche revealed his interest in madness and madmen. *Daybreak, The Gay Science,* and *Thus Spoke Zarathustra,* appearing between 1880 and 1884, all contain significant passages on Nietzsche's ideas about madness. The most famous of these is the parable of the madman seeking God with a lantern (*The Gay Science, s.* 125). However a passage more relevant to Nietzsche's own history is to be found in Section 14, Book 1 of *Daybreak.* Anyone who thinks there is a simple clinical explanation for Nietzsche's sudden plunge into psychosis would do well to reflect on it. Nietzsche later considered himself to be *the* great innovator in the history of morality. Had the memory of this passage sunk into his subconscious mind? It is given in full below (Book 1, *s*.14):

Significance of Madness in the History of Morality

When in spite of that fearful pressure of the "morality of morals" under which all the communities of mankind have lived many thousands of years before our current reckoning of time and, generally, in the same way up to the present day (we ourselves live in the little world of exceptions and as if in the evil zone): when I say, in spite of this, new and changing thoughts, valuations, drives broke out again and again, they did so within a frightening framework; almost everywhere it is madness which paved the way, which broke the spell of honored usage and superstition. Do you understand why this had to be madness? Something in voice and gesture so terrible and unpredictable as the demonic moods of the weather and the sea and therefore worthy of a similar fear and perception. Something that so visibly carried the mark of absolute compulsion like the convulsions and the foaming of the epileptic which appeared to mark the madman as mask and sounding-horn of the godhead. Something that gave to the bearer of a new idea reverence and awe of himself and spared him the pangs of conscience, driving him to become a prophet and martyr? While it is always said today that the genius, rather than a grain of salt, is given a grain of the spice of madness, all earlier peoples thought that wherever there was madness, there was also a grain of genius and wisdom, something "God-like" as one whispered to oneself. Or rather, as was expressed forcefully enough, "The greatest benefits have come to Greece through madness," which Plato said, along with the rest of antiquity. Let us go a step further: all those superior individuals who were irresistibly drawn to throw off the yoke of some moral custom and give a new law, had no alternative, *if they were not actually mad*, to make themselves mad or set themselves up as mad— and of course this refers to originators in all areas, not only to the priestly and political figures: even the originator of poetical meter had to make himself believable through madness. (A certain convention of madness was attached to poets even into much milder eras: to which, for example, Solon had recourse when he urged the Athenians to the reconquest of Salamis.) "How does one make himself mad if he is not and does not dare to appear so?"—almost all the significant men of antiquity have preoccupied themselves with this fearful idea; a secret lore of tricks and dietary signs propagate themselves beside the feeling of guiltlessness, even holiness of such ponderings and intentions. The formulas for becoming a medicine man among the Indians, a holy man among the Christians of the Middle Ages, an Angekok among Greenlanders, a pajee among Brazilians are in essence all the same: senseless fasting, continuous sexual abstinence, going into the desert or climbing a mountain or a column, or "sitting on an aged willow tree which looks out over a lake" and thinking of nothing more than that which brings with it rapture and spiritual convulsions. Who dares to cast a glance into the wilderness of the bitter and overflowing spiritual distress in which the most productive men of all times have languished! To listen to those sounds of lonely and distraught men: "Ah, then give me madness, you heavenly powers! Madness so that I can finally believe in myself! Give me delirium and convulsions, sudden light and darkness, frighten me with frost and fire as no mortal has ever felt, with din and surrounding forms, let me howl and whimper and creep like an animal: only that I may find belief in myself. Doubt consumes me, I have destroyed the law, the law frightens me like a corpse does a living person: if I am not *more* than the law then I am the most wretched of all. This new spirit in me, from whence does it come if not from you? Prove to me that I am from you; madness alone proves it to me." And only too often this fervor reaches its goal all too well: in that time when Christianity most demonstrated its fruitfulness with holy men and desert hermits, there were enormous madhouses in Jerusalem for unfortunate holy men, for those who had given up their last grain of salt.

Nietzsche had heard from Peter Gast that Turin might be a desirable place to reside. In April of 1888 he journeyed there to spend the spring. The visit had an inauspicious beginning, he took a wrong train and had to spend a night in a strange place. When he arrived in Turin, it was rainy and cold. However, from the beginning, Nietzsche had the feeling it was the perfect place for him. A letter to Gast on April 7, 1888, enumerated the reasons he liked Turin. It was not a large place, not at all modern as he had feared but redolent of a seventeenth century Renaissance town. He liked the yellow and reddish-brown architecture found throughout giving a unity of style to the central city. He particularly appreciated the flat, well-paved streets, important to a near-blind person like Nietzsche. Everything was less expensive than in the other parts of Italy where he had lived. He had found lodging with a congenial Italian family near the center of town. The cafés looked enticing to him. The bridges over the river Po were wonderfully attractive, beyond good and evil!

In June of 1888, Nietzsche traveled to Sils-Maria for his customary summer residence in Switzerland. The weather was unusually cold with a rare heavy snowfall in July. He felt worse than usual there and sent off depressing letters to Overbeck, Peter Gast, and Carl Fuchs. After three months, he returned to his old lodgings in Turin with the Fino family. There his health and state of mind changed dramatically.

6

Breakdown in Turin

Throughout his years as a wandering philosopher, Nietzsche often revealed evidence of a depressed state of mind. His letters to friends and family were filled with the most pathetic descriptions of his health, his loneliness, and his mental state. Thoughts of suicide were described on occasion. A letter to Franz Overbeck on July 4, 1888, is a typical example of the type of letter one might receive from Nietzsche:

Since I have left Turin, I've been in a miserable condition. Constant headaches, constant vomiting; a recrudescence of my old troubles; concealing of a deep nervous exhaustion in which the whole machine isn't good for anything. Or rather, I can think clearly but not favorably over my total situation. I am not only lacking health but also the precondition for becoming healthy—the life strength is no longer intact. The losses of at least 10 years can't be made good any more: I've been living off my "capital" and nothing, nothing at all has been replenished. That makes one *poor*.

Yet on his return to Turin for a second time in the fall of 1888, Nietzsche's state of mind seemed to radically change. Suddenly, everything became good for him, more than good, everything was "perfect." Turin was just the right place for him, the people there treated him sympathetically and he liked the food. He felt ten years younger, in good health, and good spirits. His work was moving forward in all directions. A letter to Overbeck on October 18 reflected his new feelings about himself:

Yesterday with your letter in my hand, I went for my customary walk outside of Turin. Purest October light everywhere; the majestic tree-lined path which led me for about an hour alongside the Po was hardly touched yet by autumn. I am the most thankful man in the world— *autumn* touched in every good sense of the word: it is my great *harvest-time*. Everything is easy for me, everything pleases me although hardly anyone could have such great things in hand as I do. That the *first* book of the *Transvaluation of all Values* is finished, ready for press, gives me a feeling for which I have no words. There will be four books; they will appear separately. This time, as an old artillerist, I am unlimbering my heavy guns: I fear I am going to smash the history of mankind into two parts.

It is not too much to use the word "euphoria," perhaps "grandiosity" to describe such a letter. Overbeck must have been amazed at the change of mood in the friend who had been such a source of concern to him.

In fact, Nietzsche was writing at a frenetic pace. Between July and November 1888, he began and completed three major works: *Twilight of the Idols, The Antichrist* and *Ecce Homo.* Nor were these casual productions; *Twilight* is an epitome of most of his significant philosophical positions, *The Antichrist* sets out his principal belief that Christianity is the source of most of the evils in European civilization and *Ecce Homo* is a unique autobiographical statement of his own tastes, habits, and interests along with a commentary on all his previously written works. Whatever one may think of the ideas expressed in these late works, there can be no doubt that the author is in full command of his mode of expression. There is no decline in organizing ability and certainly not of intelligence; it has been pointed out that his works of 1888 are more consistently theme oriented than his earlier works. One of his English translators and biographers, R.J. Hollingdale, comments that the works of 1888 represent "Nietzsche's victory over the most intractable of his opponents, the German language: the famous brevity of these last works is an effect of absolute control over the means of expression."[1] Walter Kaufmann, whose translations have made Nietzsche known to English readers, said he prefers the works of 1888 to all the other Nietzsche writings. *Ecce Homo*, wrote Kaufmann, is one of the treasures of world literature.[2]

The point of mentioning these encomiums about Nietzsche's 1888 writings is to emphasize that they could not be the work of a man suffering from an organic dementia, whatever its cause. There was a definite alteration of his mood but not of his cognitive abilities. One can characterize Nietzsche as euphoric, grandiose, perhaps even psychopathic if one takes offense at some of his ideas but in no way demented, that is to say manifesting a loss of intellectual abilities. This is a critical point when evaluating the nature of his mental disorder as it revealed itself toward the end of the year.

After Nietzsche finished *Ecce Homo* in November 1888, his drive to write became channeled into his correspondence. Although he had always been a prolific letter writer, the number of letters composed and dispatched at that time is astounding. There are well over 100 letters attributed to him during the period from mid-November to January 6, 1889, when he collapsed into frank psychosis. No doubt there are others still in private hands which have not been published. They seem to show an increasing tendency toward loss of contact with reality, although his letters to his publisher C. G. Naumann are very precise in every detail. Raoul Richter, who edited the first edition of *Ecce Homo* in 1905, described his manuscript corrections as "miniature graphic masterpieces," every letter was readable and every insertion exactly placed.[3] Apparently Nietzsche was capable of functioning at this time on two different levels of reality testing. The letters of December 31 to January 6, the so-called "madness" notes, reveal a total loss of concern with the real world. The very last letter composed by him, on January 6, 1889, was sent to Jacob Burckhardt. It is worth quoting in full because, besides revealing his mental processes at the time, it was the main factor responsible for Overbeck's Turin journey to take charge of his mentally disabled friend.

Dear Herr Professor,

In the end, I would rather be a Basel professor than God; however, I have not dared to pursue my private egotism so far so as to abandon the creation of the world. You see, one must make sacrifices where and how one lives. Yet I have a little student room reserved for myself, which is opposite the Carignano Palace (in which I was born as Victor Emmanuel), and besides permits me to hear from its work desk the splendid music from the Galleria Subalpina. I pay 25 francs with service, pay for my own tea and groceries, suffer with torn boots and thank heaven every moment for the *old* world for which men have not been simple and quiet enough. Since I am condemned to spend the next eternity making bad jokes, so I do a little writing here which really doesn't require much, very pretty and not at all demanding. The post office is five steps away, I put my own letters there in order to become the great feuilletonist of the *grande monde*. Naturally, I am in close connection with Figaro, and so that you can have an idea how inoffensive I can be, listen to my first two bad jokes:

Don't take the case of Prado too hard. I am Prado, I am also the father of Prado, I dare say I am also Lesseps . . . I want to give my Parisians whom I love a new concept—that of an upright criminal. I am also Chambige—also an upright criminal.

Second joke. I greet the immortal Monsieur Daudet belonging to the *quarante*.

Astu

What is unpleasant and adds to my modesty is that I am fundamentally every name in history; also regarding the children which I have put into the world, I have some mistrust whether everything that enters the "kingdom of God" also comes from *God*. During this autumn, lightly dressed as possible, I was twice at my gravesites, first as Count Robilant (no, that is my son, insofar as I am Carlo Alberto, in my nature here below) but I was Antonelli myself. Dear Herr Professor, you should see this edifice; since I am quite inexperienced in the things which I create, I will be grateful for any criticism you make without promising to make use of it. We artists can't be taught. Today I have seen my operetta— brilliantly Moorish—and take this opportunity to notice that now Moscow as well as Rome are grandiose affairs. You see, I am not without talent for landscapes as well. Consider it, we'll have a fine, fine chat, Turin isn't far, there aren't serious professional duties, a glass of Veltliner could be obtained. Casual dress is appropriate.

With heartfelt love your
Nietzsche

Tomorrow my son Umberto is coming with the darling Margherita who I will however receive in my shirtsleeves. The *rest* is for Frau Cosima . . . Ariadne . . . from time to time becomes entranced . . .

I go everywhere in my student jacket, slap here and there someone on the shoulder and say; *siamo contenti? son dio, ho fatto questa caricatura . . .* (are we content? I am God, I have made this caricature . . .)

I have put Caiaphas in chains, also I have been crucified by German doctors last year in a very drawn-out manner. Wilhelm Bismarck and all anti-Semites abolished.

You can make use of this letter in any manner that does not lower me in the regard of the people of Basel.

At first glance, this letter may seem to be properly categorized as a "mad" note. However, further inspection reveals that there is a logic running through the entire composition albeit the logic is uniquely Nietzsche's own requiring special interpretation. All of the names in it have a definite connection with recent experiences of Nietzsche and the bizarre, apparently mad statements have a definite foundation in concepts previously expressed by him. Verrechia provides the background details for most of the names and events mentioned.[4] Nietzsche's casual assumption of the personality of the various historical figures mentioned relates to his philosophy of the eternal return which is set forth in many of his writings, especially *Thus Spoke Zarathustra*. The first sentence in the letter bears consideration as it expresses in a remarkable manner a key aspect of Nietzsche's self-concept.

Perhaps the aspect of this letter that most reflects Nietzsche's break with reality is that he should have sent it to its recipient. Jacob Burckhardt was a former older colleague of Nietzsche's and eminent historical scholar in his own right who never was comfortable with the younger man's free-wheeling literary style. There was no empathy for Nietzschean logic in his mind. As Overbeck once exclaimed; how could he have sent such a letter to Burckhardt of all people! This missive sent to Peter Gast would have been received with delight and appreciation. Gast understood that Nietzsche "was a culture unto himself" even if he did not fully appreciate the degree to which Nietzsche was losing his footing in the real world.

In any case, Burckhardt concluded from the letter that Nietzsche was insane. He paid an unaccustomed visit to Franz Overbeck who lived nearby and whom he knew was in frequent contact with Nietzsche. Overbeck took the letter to Dr. Ludwig Wille who was the director of the Basel psychiatric clinic and who knew Nietzsche from an earlier meeting. Wille concluded that the author of the letter needed immediate psychiatric care. Correspondence would not do, Overbeck would have to immediately proceed to Turin. Thus was set in motion the sequence of events that led to Nietzsche's institutionalization.

It is necessary to back up at this point to consider Nietzsche's situation in Turin at the end of 1888. In spite of his euphoria, Nietzsche was under severe pressures from a number of sources. He felt that *Ecce Homo* had to be translated into the other major European languages in order to obtain a hearing. Besides what he felt to be the inborn incapacity of Germans to understand his work, there was a real danger it would be seized by the censor and legal action brought against him. In spite of his optimistic statements, he had made no progress in obtaining any translators for the work. His financial situation was precarious and his pension was scheduled to be cut by one-third during the following year. Because he had been forced to subsidize his own works for many years, the prospects for future publication, including translations, must have seemed very dim. Moreover, he must have realized that his last corrections of *Ecce Homo* contained statements about his mother and sister which would probably alienate them from him for a long time, if not forever. Given his diminishing circle of real friends—really only Overbeck and Peter Gast—he must have felt more isolated than ever.

The letter to Burckhardt was not the only event that had brought Overbeck to Turin. Up to this point, Nietzsche's clowning and exaggerations were confined to his literary expression, especially his letters. However, on November 25, he wrote to Peter Gast that "I make so many stupid jokes to myself and have so much private buffoonery that I sometimes spend a half hour on the street *grimacing*, I don't know any other word for it." The grimacing recurred and, after his breakdown, was repeatedly mentioned in descriptions of him. There must have been other behavioral disturbances which worried his landlord, David Fino, because he apparently arranged several visits with a Turin psychiatrist named Professor Carlo Turina.[5] The physician prescribed bromides for sedation indicating overstimulation was thought to be at least part of the problem.

It is easy to misinterpret much of what Nietzsche said and did without an understanding of the role "clowning" played in his consciousness. Back in 1882 when he was composing *The Gay Science*, the following thought appears (*s.* 153):

Homo poeta. I myself who have composed this tragedy of tragedies, as far as it is finished; I who have first bound the knot of morality into existence and tied it so tight that only a God can loosen it—as was required by Horace—I myself have destroyed all the gods in the fourth act—out of morality! What shall now become of the fifth act! From whence shall come a tragic solution!—must I begin to think about a comic solution?

Nietzsche did not forget about comic solutions to his problems. On July 18, 1888, in a letter advising Carl Fuchs that their literary friendship was being terminated (which he later retracted), Nietzsche commented:

I have given men the deepest book they possess, my Zarathustra: a book which is so exceptional that whoever can say "I have understood six sentences in it, meaning experienced" belongs to a higher order of mortals—However how one must atone for that! must pay for it! it almost ruins one's character. The cleft has become too great. Since then I really only carry on clowning (*Possenreisserei*), in order to keep control over an unbearable tension and vulnerability.

Nietzsche was accused by Ferdinand Avenarius, editor of *Kunstwart*, an arts magazine in which Nietzsche and some of his friends published letters, of descending to the level of a "Feuilletonist" in his writings. This was severe criticism, implying a lack of seriousness and a commercial motivation in a writer so labeled. Nietzsche, although by then was revealing problems with his reality testing, responded with a cogent letter to Avenarius (December 10, 1888) explaining his position about his writing style. "That the deepest spirit must also be the most frivolous, that is almost the formula for my philosophy." This attitude needs to be remembered when evaluating many of Nietzsche's more outrageous statements, particularly his political *pronunciamentos*. The formula is repeated in a slightly different context in *Beyond Good and Evil*, *s.* 223, "Perhaps it is just here where we can discover our own *invention*, the kingdom where we can still be original, as a parodist of world history and as the buffoon of God,—if nothing else today has a future, perhaps it is just our *laughter* which will still have one."

The first real evidence that Nietzsche had lost the ability to look out for himself occurred during the first week of January 1889. The conventional story is that he threw his arms around the neck of a dray horse who was being mistreated by his master and then collapsed in the street. It is not clear what really happened but what is known is that his landlord, David Fino, was nearby and was summoned to take his agitated tenant home. The police appeared to have been also involved and there was some fear that Nietzsche might be taken to a *manicomio*, the Italian version of an institution for the insane. Such a fate had occurred to other German expatriates in Italy. As usual with the events in Turin, many interesting details elaborating on Nietzsche's Turin experiences are provided by Verrechia.[6] Later, Elisabeth Förster-Nietzsche let it be known that this was the first of Nietzsche's "strokes" that contributed to his breakdown (along with overuse of drugs) but there is no reliable evidence that he suffered a stroke at this time. Afterwards Fino, probably reaching the end of his tolerance for his mentally ill tenant, found Overbeck's address and telegrammed him to come to Turin. Thus Overbeck had a double reason to make the trip.

After arriving in Turin by overnight train, Overbeck had some difficulties in finding Nietzsche's lodgings. He has provided a graphic description of how Nietzsche appeared at the time of his arrival:

I saw Nietzsche in a sofa corner, crouched down and reading—as it turned out, the last proof reading of N. contra Wagner—he looked horribly decrepit; recognizing me, he threw himself upon me and embraced me strongly, breaking into a torrent of tears, then sinking back onto the sofa. I too could hardly stand upright from the shock. Had he at this moment recognized the abyss opening in front of him or in which he was actually plunged? In any case, the moment did not return. The whole family Fino was present. Scarcely had he started moaning and quivering again when he was given some bromine water that stood on the table. In a moment, he was calm again and smiling, he began to speak of the great reception that was prepared for the evening. So he was in the grip of delusional ideas which never left while I was with him. He broke forth into loud singing and frenzied piano playing, fragments out of the mental world in which he had been recently living and interspersed with indescribably uttered expressions, sublime, wonderfully insightful and unspeakably horrible things about himself as the successor to a dead God, all punctuated by chords from the piano after which convulsions and outbursts of unspeakable suffering followed—yet as I have said, these occurred only for brief moments when I was there; in general, they were outweighed by the profession of his vocation to be the comic character of the new eternity, although he, the incomparable master of expression, was incapable of expressing the rapture of his happiness other than with trivial expressions or comical dancing and jumping. At the same time, the childish inoffensiveness never left him even during the three nights during which his outbursts kept the whole household awake. Just this inoffensiveness and his almost unconditional docility as soon as one entered into his ideas of royal receptions, arrangements, festivals and so forth made it child's play, at least for the attendant which I had on Wille's insistence found in Turin, to arrange the transportation [to Basel].[7]

There were a few memories that Overbeck left out of his letter to Peter Gast. More personal details were revealed later in intimate conversations.[8] It appears that Nietzsche danced naked, evoking the antique conception of holy sexual frenzies. Overbeck might not have read *The Gay Science*, or if he had, he might have forgotten passage *s*. 381 where Nietzsche says, "I don't know what the spirit of a philosopher would wish for more than to be a good dancer. The dance is really his ideal, also his art, and in the end, his unique piety, his 'service to God.' " One could hardly expect Overbeck to maintain a philosophic calm in the face of a case like Nietzsche's. However, reading Overbeck's agitated account, it seems clear that Nietzsche's mind was still working although dominated by his own unique logic and ideas. What is more ominous than his outbursts and delusional ideas is the "docility" (*Harmloskeit*) with which he allowed himself to be moved about and manipulated. His volitional sense was disintegrating, this more than anything else was probably responsible for his final decay.

The next day, Overbeck, Dr. Bettman who had been hired for the trip, and Nietzsche left the lodgings for the train trip home. Nietzsche did not want to get out of bed, surely he had a premonition of what lay ahead. But Dr. Bettman cajoled him into leaving through promises of receptions, pageants, and the like. It is not likely that Nietzsche was fooled but his capacity for independent decision was gone and he went along with the charade. He was given chloral hydrate for the trip so that he slept much of the time. However, when he was awake, Overbeck heard him singing what he described as a wonderful song with a strange melody. It was the Venetian Gondola song, one of the last poems that Nietzsche wrote, which he inserted in both *Ecce Homo* and *Nietzsche contra Wagner*. The last stanza is reproduced below:

> My soul, a stringed instrument
> invisibly touched,
> sang secretly to itself
> a Gondola song,
> trembling with an iridescent bliss.
> —Was anyone listening? . . .

The little group arrived at the Basel train station in the early morning where a waiting cab took them to Friedmatt, the Basel psychiatric clinic headed by Dr. Wille. There were no further difficulties with the trip. Nietzsche spent the next fourteen months as an institutional patient.

During the last six weeks of 1888, Nietzsche developed a lively correspondence with August Strindberg, the notorious Swedish genius. There was a mutual admiration between them, based no doubt, in large part on similarities in their outlooks on life. Strindberg also manifested many psychotic features in his personality but he was a tougher character than Nietzsche and managed to escape the institutions. Nietzsche wanted him to translate *Ecce Homo* into French but Strindberg did not encourage their business relationship saying his fee would probably be too high for the impoverished Nietzsche. Strindberg received one of Nietzsche's "madness" notes which was signed "Nietzsche Caesar." However Strindberg was not one to be taken aback by either clowning or madness. The response, although somewhat mad itself, shows a deep perception of Nietzsche's personality. The letter is written mostly in Latin quoting Horace. The first line written by Strindberg in Greek derives from Anacreon.

Dearest Doctor:
   "I will, I will be raving mad!"
   I could not read your letter without a severe shock and I thank you very much.

"You would lead a better life, Licinius, if you neither shaped your life constantly toward the open sea, nor, shivering tremulously in the face of the storm, held too closely to the treacherous coast."

Meanwhile let us rejoice in our madness.

Fare you well and remain true to your

Strindberg (Deus, optimus maximus)[9]

It was unfortunate that Strindberg's advice came too late for Nietzsche to consider. As he said in one of his last letters to Peter Gast (December 31, 1888), he had crossed the Rubicon and no longer knew his address.

Asylum Inmate

Nietzsche's little party was greeted by Dr. Wille at the entry area of Friedmatt, the mental institution directed by Wille. Overbeck thought that Nietzsche had no idea of where he was and was fearful what might happen when Nietzsche learned the truth of his circumstances. However, Nietzsche in his most urbane manner approached Wille directly saying he knew he had seen him before but could not recollect his name. "I am Wille" was the response. In the calmest of tones, Nietzsche responded, "Wille? You are an asylum doctor (*Irrenarzt*). I had a conversation with you some years ago about religious delusions. The occasion was an insane person, Adolf Vischer who lived here or in Basel at the time." Wille listened silently and nodded in agreement. Overbeck was amazed at Nietzsche's detailed recollection of events occurring seven years ago but also of his complete denial that he himself was now the patient of an *Irrenarzt*. It was another example, as Overbeck himself put it, "of the annihilating split in his personality."[1]

Nietzsche allowed himself to be handed over to the care of an assistant physician without difficulty. He was to have breakfast and a bath, and then be conducted to his room. Initially he was obedient and obliging. He ate breakfast ravenously, enjoyed his bath afterwards. An examination was then performed by the assistant physician. The details are all available at the present time in the Nietzsche Archives and have been published.[2] There are few pertinent points to be noted from the physical examination. Nietzsche was described as a healthy well-developed man. The asymmetries of his pupils and their slowness to react to light were described. There was no retinal examination and Nietzsche's history of chorioretinitis and lifelong pupillary asymmetry were not available to the Basel physicians. Various minor neurological signs of little importance were described. The absence of tremor or speech disorder was specifically noted. In contrast to the physical examination, his mental state was markedly abnormal. A constant flow of speech was noted, often confused and without logical connection. He sang and joked intermittently. He did not seem to know where he was. It was noted that he said he had "infected" himself twice which was taken to mean he had contracted syphilitic infections.

On the side of the page containing the medical history, there was a category entitled *Illness*. The entry inserted there read "Progressive paralysis" (general paresis). It was later demonstrated by Verrechia that the handwriting of that entry was that of Dr. Wille and had been added later. The diagnosis must have been made on the basis of Nietzsche's mental disorder (the "classic" psychotic megalomania), the pupillary findings, and the history of syphilis. Wille himself was said to be an authority on general paresis with many such cases at his institution. Nevertheless, it was a surprising diagnosis to make with minimal neurological signs and after only one week of observation.

Nietzsche's eight days in Friedmatt were characterized by alternating manic excitement and sleeping as a consequence of sulfonal administration. At times he would converse quite normally but then lapse into confused delusional thoughts or singing and joking. According to a later communication by Wille to Elisabeth Förster-Nietzsche, there was considerable erotic ideation in his flight of ideas. He continued to express a euphoric state of mind in which he felt strong, healthy, lucky, and capable of anything. It was noted that he would be calm while he was confined to his bed, but upon rising, the wild excitement would return. However, on balance, it was thought that the manic behavior was gradually decreasing during his stay at Friedmatt.[3]

Nietzsche's mother wanted to take her son home to Naumburg.

She was convinced that under her ministrations, he could become well again. However, Wille believed this to be inadvisable and would not agree to discharge Nietzsche to his mother's care. Finally, a compromise was worked out; Nietzsche would be transferred to the state psychiatric institution at Jena, which was only a short distance from Naumburg. The head of the Jena asylum, Professor Otto Binswanger, a well-known figure in German psychiatric circles, agreed to accept Nietzsche as a patient. On January 17, he left Basel in the company of his mother, an attendant from the Basel institution, and a young doctor named Ernst Mähly who had been a former student of Nietzsche's. He is described as leaving the institution at night, "closely flanked by both escorts, silent, his face like a mask, and in an unnaturally stiff posture, Nietzsche climbed into the train."[4] He was quiet during the first part of the trip, eating rolls his mother provided and reading newspapers with interest. However, shortly before arriving in Frankfurt where a change of trains was required, Nietzsche fell into a rage, apparently directed against his mother.[5] It was necessary for her to complete the trip in another compartment. In the absence of Frau Nietzsche, no further information exists on the rest of his journey.

There are a few points of interest about Dr. Mähly, one of Nietzsche's escorts. He was a great admirer of Nietzsche's, considering him to have been one of the great figures of German literature who had fallen in desperate straits. He was also a friend of Dr. Wille and undoubtedly familiar with the diagnosis made in Basel as to the cause of Nietzsche's condition. He and the attendant brought their patient into the Jena asylum from the railroad station. Knowing professional courtesies of physicians, one may assume that the diagnosis was communicated to the Jena staff. A full copy of the Basel medical records was not sent to Jena until some months later but Dr. Mähly undoubtedly made the gist of the information available to them on delivery of the patient. In later years, Mähly committed suicide; his father attributed his unhappy end to the evil influence of Nietzsche.

Nietzsche was an inmate in the Jena institution for fourteen months. It was the period during which his mental disorder became consolidated, whatever the cause one attributes to it. In order to understand Nietzsche's environment at that time, consideration needs to be given to the state of German psychiatry during that period, to the nature of the Jena institution, and to the background of its director, Professor Otto Binswanger. The attitudes toward Nietzsche's illness and the care which he received were greatly determined by these factors.

Psychiatry in Europe at the dawn of the nineteenth century was being transformed by attitudes of psychiatrists whose minds were formed by the ideals of the French Revolution. The painting by Fleury in 1795 of the famous Dr. Pinel freeing the mental patients of the Saltpêtrière from their chains symbolized the attitude of the times. Mental illness was thought to be due to uncontrolled passions, moral weakness or evil outside influences. Moral reeducation was the means for correcting these problems. It was an essentially humanistic view of psychiatric care. However, these views soon gave way to a different approach to mental illnesses, a view that saw them as manifestations of diseases of the brain. More than any other nineteenth century figure, this view was propagated by Dr. Wilhelm Griesinger (1817–1869). Griesinger, initially a professor at Zurich, transformed the old asylum into a university clinic whose dominant theme was not moral reeducation, but determination of the nature of brain disease causing mental illness. His textbook titled *Mental Pathology and Therapeutics*, first published in 1845, was highly influential in the field for many years. Later he became professor of psychiatry and medicine at the University of Berlin, becoming the first full-time university professor of psychiatry. As part of his emphasis on the brain as the central focus of psychiatrists, he tried to unify psychiatry, neurology, and neuropathology and focused their field of action in the university scientific scene. He succeeded to a great extent in this effort, making Germany the foremost locale for the pursuit of scientific psychiatry.

The state-supported mental institution at Jena was developed with the ideals of Griesinger very much in mind. It was closely affiliated with the University of Jena so that Binswanger could be at the same time professor of psychiatry and director of the institution. There were facilities for microscopic and experimental work; the performance of postmortem studies was an important part of German psychiatry at the time. Its facilities for patient care were thought to be representative of the most modern approaches in institutional care, embodying a pavilion system where different classes of patients could be separated into different areas. Patients were allowed considerable freedom when possible. There was regular clinical instruction conducted on a daily basis, presumably for medical students and advanced trainees. All in all, it embodied all the principles of modern scientific psychiatry as it was understood in the latter half of the nineteenth century.[6]

Otto Binswanger (1852–1929), director of the institution, possessed all credentials necessary for his prestigious post. His father, Ludwig Binswanger, had been the director of the psychiatric division of a Swiss canton hospital and founder of Kuranstalt Bellevue, a well-known mental institution in Germany. Otto had studied medicine in Heidelberg, Strassburg, and Zurich, after which he spent several years in neuropathological research in Vienna and Göttingen. He then chose psychiatry as his specialty, working as a chief physician under the well-known neuropsychiatrist Carl Westphal. (Westphal later became insane and was treated for a period of time in the Jena institution.) Finally in 1882, when not quite 30 years of age, Otto Binswanger was appointed to his twin posts as director of the Jena institution and professor of psychiatry at the University of Jena. He spent the remainder of his professional career in these posts.

In early 1889, when Nietzsche was admitted to the Jena institution, Binswanger was entering into the height of his academic career. A flow of publications was beginning in the form of scientific articles, conference presentations, textbook chapters, and editing of manuals of psychiatry. Some of his titles are given by Volz[7]; "Brain syphilis and dementia paralytica, clinical and statistical studies," "Teaching Psychiatric Clinics," "The Pathological Histology of Cortical Damage in General Progressive Paralysis with Special Attention to Acute and Early Forms," "The Delineation of General Progressive Paralysis," "Contributions to the Pathogenesis and Differential Diagnosis of Progressive Paralysis," "Pathology and Therapy of Neurasthenia." There were many others as well as coauthorship of a textbook titled *Textbook of Psychiatry* that underwent several editions. Progressive paralysis was his area of special expertise.

Besides his research and publications, Binswanger carried a substantial teaching load. He gave lectures three times weekly on subjects such as clinic for mental disorders, spinal cord disorders and "nervousness." One special topic of his was "pathological-histological work in the laboratory" revealing his personal interest in neuropathology, a subject which will again be discussed in conjunction with the absence of postmortem examination of Nietzsche. A vivid example of his teaching style is described by a former medical student who was present during a case presentation by Binswanger of none other than—Professor Nietzsche! Nietzsche was exhibited to the class as an example of general paresis. Binswanger has been criticized by some subsequent writers for putting Nietzsche on public view in this manner but this was and still is standard practice in medical education.

Binswanger is a typical example of the medical academician who pursues a wide variety of academic activities requiring research, teaching, and administration. The type has changed little over the years. He could not have had much time for prolonged attention to patients, not to speak of focusing on an unusual personality such as Nietzsche. The era of psychoanalysis had not yet arrived. When Frau Nietzsche gave him *Nietzsche contra Wagner* to read, he responded by saying he had little time for "belles lettres" (*Schöngeisterschriften*). He did read the one-paragraph preface which appeared to him to be "fearfully excited." Later, when Nietzsche had become famous, he became more acquainted with Nietzsche's books and was presented with a bound collection of his works by Frau Nietzsche.

Although Nietzsche was listed as Binswanger's private patient, the initial examination was conducted and recorded by Dr. Theodor Ziehen, the chief house physician who later went on to become a well-known psychiatrist and author of a major textbook of psychiatry. All of the brief notes during his fourteen-month stay were made by various assistant staff physicians. Only some historical details about Nietzsche were recorded by Binswanger himself, presumably largely on the basis of information provided by Dr. Mähly on admission or possibly by the mother because Nietzsche himself was in no condition to provide any kind of reliable history about his own background. Binswanger's notes include the statement, "Medical history from Basel" although the complete Basel record did not reach Jena until later in the year. Perhaps Mähly provided a written clinical summary. It is noteworthy that the Jena admission form carries the entry—*Type of Illness: Paralytic mental illness.*[8] Evidently the Basel diagnosis was carried over to Jena without alteration. The initial evaluation gave the physicians no reason to change this diagnosis.

The examination at Jena was essentially similar to Basel, although there are more technical details of the examination given which add little to the total picture. A "scar" on the penis was noted which has been taken by some to indicate prior syphilis although this is a totally unjustifiable assumption.[9] The pupillary asymmetries are noted. Speech again is noted to be essentially normal, handwriting shows tremor "when upset." Reading abilities were normal. The major findings, as in Basel, were connected with his mental state and behavior. He thanked the attendants for his "splendid reception." He did not seem to know where he was. At times he seemed to think he was in Naumburg, at times in Turin. He gesticulated a great deal and chattered continuously, often in French or Italian. (It was noted that in spite of his long residence in Italy, he did not know much Italian.) He continually tried to shake the hand of his doctor. Regarding the content of his "flight of ideas," he spoke of his musical compositions and sang excerpts from them, he claimed to have counseled "legations" and to have given service to them. During his speech, he grimaced almost continuously. Even at night he engaged in almost continuous disconnected chatter. Today the patient would be said to be in a state of obvious manic psychosis. The Jena records have been reproduced by Volz with relevant comments of Nietzsche's physicians, family, and friends.[10]

The principal concern of the Jena physicians was to reduce the level of his excitement. "Calm, calm and always more calm" was Binswanger's invariable prescription to the mother when she was responsible for his care. To this end, Frau Nietzsche was not permitted to visit her son in the institution until July 29, over six months after his admission. She received regular reports, however, from Dr. Ziehen and an acquaintance, Frau Gelzer, who had information about Nietzsche's condition in the institution. For the first months of Nietzsche's commitment, he continued to exhibit agitated and incoherent behavior on frequent occasions. There was smearing of feces and drinking of urine, facts which were omitted on the first publications of the Jena record. At times he had to be isolated because of agitated behavior. Episodes were reported which suggest erotic or persecutory delusions; for example, on April 1 he told the warder "24 whores were with me at night"; April 17—"the most fearful machinery has been turned against me"; and April 19—"I want a revolver if the suspicion is true that the Grandduke himself has committed these *Schweinerei* and attacks against me." On June 6, he broke a window in his agitation. Frau Nietzsche wrote to Overbeck's wife that she had learned that when Professor Binswanger and his wife sat in their garden (he lived on the grounds), they could always hear Nietzsche's loud voice. But on other occasions, he could be quite reasonable, respond sensibly to questions, recognize his physicians and know where he was, and discuss his family.[11]

By June, he seemed calmer and was able to take daily walks on the grounds. He occasionally read the newspapers, seemingly understanding what he read and remembering their contents at a later date. He often complained of headaches, reminiscent of his earlier problem with migraine. While there were still intermittent behavioral lapses (smearing feces, grimacing, urinating in his water glass), his overall condition had sufficiently improved so that his mother was permitted a visit on July 29, 1889. She had not seen him since the transport to Jena in mid-January of that year. By and large, the visit went well, Nietzsche seemed pleased to see her. There was no recurrence of the rage reaction directed against her during the trip to Jena.

During this time, he received a mercury treatment in the form of "inunctions," a rubbing-in of the medication. Even in those days it was not thought to be effective in general paresis but the treatment seemed to be a favorite of Dr. Ziehen. On August 16, there was reported the closest thing to a visual hallucination noted during his illness; he broke a window because he thought he saw a rifle behind it. Although his behavior was calmer, he still often gave evidence of incoherence and loss of contact with reality. A letter written by Professor Binswanger to Overbeck on September 23, 1889, summarized his condition nine months after his admission.

Regarding the condition of Herr Professor Nietzsche, we can see that there is a clear improvement since he speaks more coherently and outbursts with screaming, etc. are less frequent. Delusions still appear intermittently as do auditory hallucinations. The attacks of weakness have not progressed and are not significant. He only partially recognizes his surroundings, for example he repeatedly refers to the chief warder as Prince Bismarck, etc. He does not exactly know who he is. He often has distinct consciousness of illness, he particularly complains of headaches.

He eats regularly but sleep is often disturbed. His mother visits him often: he recognizes her immediately and speaks quite intelligibly with her; also he remembers such visits quite well the next day. He still soils himself. The outlook for recovery is small, however not completely impossible. We will be able to make a definite judgment about his course during the next three months.[12]

Binswanger was very cautious in this statement. His refusal to give a clearly negative prognosis is hard to understand in view of the diagnosis which has been made and the prevailing medical belief at the time that progressive paralysis was uniformly fatal within a few years. Binswanger was an authority on the condition, familiar with its accepted prognosis. It indicates a degree of uncertainty about the diagnosis even after nine months of observation.

In December 1889, an eccentric individual named Julius Langbehn who professed himself to be a disciple of Nietzsche began taking daily walks with him. He claimed he would be able to cure Nietzsche through aggressively confronting him with Christian doctrine, an odd idea considering the consistently anti-Christian view expressed in Nietzsche's writings. There is general agreement that Langbehn was a strange figure who was unlikely to contribute anything to improving Nietzsche's mental condition. However, some of Langbehn's observations about Nietzsche's situation in the Jena institution are worth considering:

He [Nietzsche] is treated in Binswanger's institution as a depraved professor, bummed-out and having become crazy in Italy, *ach nein*, not as a professor but as an imprisoned person; such treatment to a person with Nietzsche's sensibilities, if he were not already ill, would destroy him: nothing of observation, of study of a sick person, nothing of the so-called modern science, which we outsiders so much respect, only a quite clumsy, unworthy and negligent dealing with a sick person! Warders who seize him and deal with him mockingly, while he knows just what is happening and feels it all as cruel and frightening. In short, Nietzsche is in a poorhouse—nothing more.[13]

Langbehn's remarks were later ignored because his criticisms were thought to be motivated by his desire to remove Nietzsche from the institution and take charge of the treatment himself. However, reading the curt entries of the hospital record and finding no evidence of any therapeutic approach to Nietzsche as a personality in his own right makes one wonder whether there was some merit in Langbehn's observations.

Nietzsche's condition was stable during his last months at the Jena institution. He was allowed to take walks with his mother and other visitors were permitted. His old friends Peter Gast and Franz Overbeck visited him during this time and both of them spent hours walking with him. Their observations show considerable perceptiveness, revealing much more about his thought processes than the terse factual entries in the medical record. Gast visited Nietzsche on January 21, 1890. It was the first time they had seen each other in over two years. Gast described the visit:

He did not look very bad. I would almost like to say his mental disturbance consists only of an accentuation of the humorous side he formerly displayed when among friends in an intimate circle. He knew me at once, embraced and kissed me and was very delighted to see me, gave me his hand again and again as though he could not believe that I was really there. We spoke much of Venice and what was very surprising to me was that he had, of all things, remembered many of my more burlesque observations.[14]

Later, Gast listened to Nietzsche play the piano. He was amazed at his capacity to improvise, to produce a mood of "Tristan-like finesse." However, Gast's optimism did not last as he spent more time with the patient. He became depressed by his recognition that the old independent Nietzsche was no longer to be found. He began to feel that his friend did not want to recover, that he "would be about as grateful to his rescuers as somebody who has jumped into the water to drown himself and has been pulled out by some fool of a coastguard." He wondered if Nietzsche was in a state which seemed to him "horrible to say—as though he were only pretending to be insane, as though he were glad to have ended this way!"[15]

Overbeck also spent long hours with Nietzsche during these last months at the Jena institution. He marveled how he could be completely lucid at one moment with even flashes of brilliancy recalling his highest moments but then suddenly sink into the most confused fantasies. He was particularly struck how childishly compliant Nietzsche had become most of the time. Like Gast, Overbeck wondered if Nietzsche was simulating madness. "I cannot escape the horrible suspicion that arises within me at certain definite periods of observation, or at least at certain moments, namely, that his madness is simulated. This impression can only be explained by the general experiences which I have had of Nietzsche's self-concealment, of his spiritual masks. But here, too, I have bowed to facts which overrule all personal thoughts and speculations."[16] Basically, Overbeck found no reason to alter the opinion he had expressed on January 17, 1889, after he had said good-bye to Nietzsche at the train station on his way to Jena—"It is all over with him."

As Nietzsche steadily improved with respect to tractability, Frau Nietzsche rented an apartment in Jena in order to be with her son daily. He spent much of each day with her either on walks or in her apartment. His mother was pleased that he was improving so much, but Peter Gast, who had remained in Jena, wrote: "Nietzsche is but a mockery of his old self! My eyes fill with tears when I think of it."[17] The crusader for spiritual independence had become childishly docile. At no time did he ever refer in a meaningful manner to his former literary ambitions. The one feature of his old self which remained was his improvisations on the piano which were marked, according to Gast, by a remarkable profundity of expression. This did not carry over, however, into his personal interchanges.

The following extract from Podach may serve to epitomize the transformation that had occurred in Nietzsche. The Gelzer family were old friends from his Basel days who were then living in Jena. Mother and son often visited them. A relation of the Gelzers who was then a young student in Jena recalled the visits:

When Frau Pastor Nietzsche wanted to visit the Gelzers she brought her son with her who ran after her like a child. So as to be undisturbed, she took him into the drawing-room where he remained standing at the door. She went to the piano and played a few chords, whereupon he came closer, and at last began to play, himself standing at first, until his mother pushed him down on the chair, if I may say so. Whereupon he would improvise for hours on end. Frau Pastor knew that her son was safe without having to look after him as long as she heard the piano.[18]

Nietzsche was discharged from the Jena institution on March 24, 1890, to the care of his mother. Some months later they returned to the family home in Naumburg where he had lived as a child before departing to Pforta. His physicians and admirers at the time regarded Frau Nietzsche as the epitome of a self-sacrificing mother who utterly devoted herself to the care of her sick son. This may be true but it is necessary to examine another side of Nietzsche's relationship with his mother in order to fully evaluate the meaning of the situation into which he was thrust. This is given in the last modifications he made to *Ecce Homo*, just before his collapse into psychosis. These changes were suppressed by his sister who came into possession of the manuscript before its publication. They have only recently come to light through the efforts of the Nietzsche scholar Mazzino Montinari and are now included in the definitive *Kritische Studienausgabe* edition of *Ecce Homo* (Why I Am So Wise, s.3):

And here I touch on the question of race. I am a Polish nobleman pur sang [an assertion often made by Nietzsche], without one drop of bad blood, least of all German blood. If I look for the profoundest opposite type to me, an incalculable vulgarity of instinct, there I always find my mother and sister; to believe myself related to such canaille would be a blasphemy against my divinity. The treatment that I experience from my mother and sister, right up to this present moment, instills me with an unspeakable horror: here operates with infallible sureness an absolute hellish machine which knows where to inflict bloody wounds, during my highest moments . . . since at those times I lack the strength to fend off poisonous worms . . . the physiological contiguity allows such a *disharmonia praestabilita* . . . however I confess that the strongest objection to the "eternal recurrence," my own profoundest thought, is always my mother and sister.[19]

Nietzsche's prose style is beginning to fall off here as the madness takes hold but the meaning is clear and there is no reason to doubt its fundamental validity. Many years later, investigators of schizophrenic disorders found prognosis to be worse when emotional overinvolvement existed with relatives of patients returning to their families.[20]

8

Descent into Apathy

From March 1890 until mid-1897, Nietzsche was cared for by his mother; after her death, his sister assumed the responsibility until the day of his physical death on August 25, 1900. For the first months after his discharge from the institution, mother and son stayed in Jena to be close to the physicians. Long walks were taken every day, initiating what Frau Nietzsche later called her *Spaziergehen-Existenz*—the walking life. Every day she would take Nietzsche walking for hours on end. She knew that he had been an inveterate walker during his independent years and hoped that return to this activity might reinvigorate his mental status. Usually he followed her about quite obediently but on occasion, especially if a stranger would approach them, he would again exhibit agitated outbursts. Finally, these behaviors came to the attention of Dr. Ziehen who warned her that if they continued, Nietzsche might have to return to the institution. This greatly frightened Frau Nietzsche, she hastily packed their belongings and returned to the family home in Naumburg.

Initially, while in Naumburg, Nietzsche's condition was relatively stable.[1] Frau Nietzsche spent virtually all her time caring for him, being helped only by her elderly housekeeper Alwine. They took daily long walks in Naumburg, often visiting the baths by the Saale river. She continued to hope for his recovery although

Professor Binswanger, who occasionally examined him in Jena, had settled on the opinion that Nietzsche's prognosis was hopeless. She read out loud to him, a practice that dated from early times when his eye problems prohibited reading on his own. Sometimes he would take up the reading himself, although there was no evidence that he was interested in what he read aloud. The Nietzsche of the era prior to institutionalization had disappeared, never again to reemerge.

By 1893, the fact that his condition was steadily deteriorating became evident to everyone who observed him. Physically, he appeared quite well and was able to continue walking for long periods, but his mother finally ceased taking him outside the home because of her anxiety about his outbursts. Walks then were limited to the veranda of the home. Mentally, however, he was rapidly sinking into apathy. He no longer recognized anyone other than his mother and Alwine. Frau Nietzsche wrote down the sayings of her son during this time which revealed a mass of cryptic, disconnected thoughts revealing the depth of Nietzsche's descent into mental vacuity. He could repeat the same sentence for hours on end. She tried to stimulate his mind through references to his former classical studies with little result. An odd feature of his talk was his tendency to use the first person when referring to mother or sister, a confusion of self highly characteristic of schizophrenic disorders. Hayman points out that when referring to his sister Elisabeth, "the insane ventriloquism is unambivalently hostile."[2] There is evidence that he had some insight into his condition, since he signed postcards (which he would write on the urgings of his mother) as *The Fool* or *The Lunatic*.

In 1894, his old friend Erwin Rohde visited him in Naumburg. Rohde was shocked by his appearance:

He is completely unresponsive, recognizes no one besides his mother and sister; bodily, he is quite shrunken, having become weak and small, aside from a healthy complexion. In short, he is a tearful sight. However, he obviously suffers no longer, no happiness or unhappiness; in some kind of fearful manner he is "beyond" everything.[3]

Meanwhile, even during his stay in the Jena institution, articles and discussions began to appear in the press about the unfortunate philosopher whose mind had suddenly broken down through overwork. Sales of his books greatly increased and appeared in local libraries. Correspondingly, the flow of royalties from his publisher also increased, more than making up for the discontinuance of the Basel pension. His sister Elisabeth Förster, whose activities in her husband's German colonization scheme in Paraguay had ended after his suicide,[4] transferred her formidable energies to her brother's literary estate. She founded the Nietzsche Archives that played an important role in making her brother known to the world at large. All during this time, Nietzsche knew nothing of his fame, vegetating in a regressed state while the long sought after recognition became a reality. At the time of his death in 1900, he was a world-renowned figure, venerated by many as the prophet of the future.

Frau Nietzsche died in 1897, apparently of a gastrointestinal cancer. She had completely devoted the last nine years of her life to the care of her mentally ill son. In so doing, she became a symbol of the unstinting devotion of a mother to her child and to the Nietzsche cults which emerged, a figure analogous to that of the Virgin Mary. Professor Binswanger continuously praised the care she gave Nietzsche, attributing his relatively healthy appearance and his very slow decline to the meticulous care provided to him by his mother. Whether the influence of the mother, taking a broad view of the situation, was really beneficial to Nietzsche is difficult to estimate. Although she was a paragon of virtue with respect to his physical needs, it is possible, as mentioned in the preceding chapter, that her continuous presence was a detrimental factor toward any possibility of regaining his pre-illness personality. Prior to the breakdown, Nietzsche had regarded her a negative influence on his literary vocation. She had no sympathy with his ambitions or comprehension of his achievements. Nevertheless, in his hour of need, she was there for him; this is perhaps the main thing which should be remembered about Frau Nietzsche.

Elisabeth Förster-Nietzsche (she reassumed her maiden name after the suicide of her husband in Paraguay) took over the responsibility for her brother after the mother's death. Actually, she had arranged for legal transfer of her brother's estate to herself even before the death of Frau Nietzsche. She was the principal representative of Nietzsche to the outside world for 40 years until her own death in 1935. A considerable literature exists documenting the ways in which she manipulated and falsified many aspects of Nietzsche's life and works. She was sympathetic to the National Socialist movement in Germany; Hitler attended her funeral in 1935 and permitted a photograph of himself next to Nietzsche's bust in Weimar. Perhaps she has become excessively demonized as a result of the reaction against her efforts to create an image of Nietzsche which suited her own interests. Nevertheless, it is hard to sympathize in any way with the ruthless control she exerted over her brother's unique literary contributions.

After the mother's death in 1897, Elisabeth transferred the entire household, including the Nietzsche Archives, to Weimar where she felt her brother's work could be better publicized. By this time, Nietzsche was little more than a breathing corpse—confined to his chair, mute, totally unresponsive to the world around him. Only occasional groans or a brief nod or shake of the head revealed there was still life in his body. He could only eat and attend to his biological functions. Yet there was something about his appearance that often created a sense of awe in visitors. Ernst Horneffer, one of the individuals working with Nietzsche's literary remains, described his impressions of the philosopher in 1899:

Nietzsche lay on a sofa, wrapped in a loose white coat—I always saw him only in this coat which heightened his prophetic appearance—and the impression was powerful, indeed overpowering. I had pictured Nietzsche quite differently. I did not find the brooding, mordantly ironic Nietzsche of the sharp, cutting aphorisms. This was another Nietzsche whom I saw there, a prophet of divine simplicity, nothing fancy in his being, in a word: the Zarathustra Nietzsche. I stood still, awestricken with reverence. The first thing I saw was the forehead, the mighty forehead. There was something Goethean, Jupiter-like in its form, and yet delicate fineness in the temples. Peter Gast says that Nietzsche did not make this Jupiter-like impression in his healthy days. That is certainly strange! As a healthy man, Nietzsche's demeanor was so modest and shy that the idea of anything very extraordinary and high did not occur. With the illness, however, consciousness disappeared, and therewith the denial of his own greatness. No visitor could escape the impression of greatness which the patient made.[5]

Dr. Ziehen visited Nietzsche in Weimar in 1898. It was the first time he had seen him since his departure from the institution. He is reported to have been surprised at Nietzsche's appearance, stating that the clinical condition of his former patient was completely different than that which would be expected with general paresis.[6] However, he did not alter his opinion that Nietzsche was suffering with this disease and that his condition was incurable.

It was about this time that Elisabeth had considered obtaining a consultation from the famous Professor Emil Kraepelin of Heidelberg. The consultation would have been very expensive and Elisabeth finally decided to ask Dr. Ziehen to see Nietzsche again as a considerably cheaper alternative. It is unfortunate that Kraepelin did not have the opportunity to examine Nietzsche. It would have been most interesting to have had his opinion about Nietzsche's illness. At this point, however, Nietzsche had so far regressed that it would have been impossible to ascertain the cause of his illness. He had slipped into the end stage of total mental deterioration, *Blödsinn*, the final common path of a variety of mental disorders which Kraepelin described so well in his authoritative textbook of psychiatry.

In the summer of 1898, the patient exhibited a sudden setback that his sister diagnosed as a "slight stroke." Another, more severe episode occurred in May 1899 which Elisabeth again diagnosed as a stroke (*Schlaganfall*). It is not clear whether these episodes were strokes in the modern sense of the term. No frank one-sided paralysis was observed afterwards nor was there any sudden change in the tempo of his regression. Nietzsche was so deteriorated by this time that it would have been hard to assess any subtle changes. It is possible that these episodes were seizures since Nietzsche himself once alluded to the possibility that he had seizures at a young age. However, these are no more than speculations, it is impossible to determine the nature of these events during this late stage of his illness. It would not be surprising, however, that a man in his mid-50s, having been bedridden for several years, should have exhibited cerebrovascular accidents, otherwise known as strokes or apoplexy. "Apoplexy" was a common diagnosis throughout the nineteenth century.

During the month of August 1900, Nietzsche developed a cold which progressed into pneumonia—again, Elisabeth's diagnosis. According to her, he again suffered a stroke, lapsing into unconsciousness. He recovered consciousness after a short period and appeared to be improving. But then his breathing became labored and "gently, without a struggle, with a last solemn, questioning look, he closed his eyes forever." She was apparently at his bed-side during his final moments. He was seven weeks short of his 56th birthday.

Elisabeth arranged an elaborate funeral ceremony with the main oration delivered by an eminent art-historian, Curt Breysig from Berlin. He is said to have spoken at inordinate length. Fritz Schu-macher, the literary worker quoted earlier with respect to Nietz-sche's appearance during his last years, comments in his reminiscences: "The same sterile scholasticism Nietzsche had always fought followed him to his grave. If he could have arisen, he would have thrown the lecturer out of the window and chased the rest of us out of his temple."[7] His body was transported two days later to Röcken to be buried in the family grave sites.

From a medical viewpoint, the most significant thing about Nietzsche's death was the absence of a postmortem examination. It is difficult to understand why this did not occur. As noted pre-viously, Binswanger had received special training in neuropa-thology and was proud of the fact that his institution possessed special facilities for microscopic studies of the brain. In 1893, he published a work titled *The Pathological Histology of Cerebral Cortex Involvement in General Paresis with Special Attention to Acute and Early Forms.*[8] The data for this study must have been being accu-mulated at about the time of Nietzsche's death, indicating that the facilities for such study continued to be available in the Jena in-stitution. Binswanger maintained excellent relations with the Nietzsche family throughout the decade after his discharge from Jena and Dr. Gutjahr, the Nietzsche family physician, maintained close contact with him during this period, presumably to benefit from his expertise about management of general paresis. Weimar was only a short distance from Jena, closer than Nietzsche's burial site in Röcken. All the conditions existed for obtaining a post-mortem study after Nietzsche's death.

Furthermore, there was considerable incentive for postmortem study, given Binswanger's status as an authority in the field of general paresis studies. Nietzsche's case was an unusual one in that he survived much longer than the three to four years after onset of major symptoms which was generally thought to be the outer limit of survival in this disease. Later Ziehen was to say that the case of Nietzsche taught the medical profession something new about general paresis, namely that occasional patients survived longer than expected. In 1890, pathological studies were the only means of confirming a diagnosis of syphilitic brain disease, much as is the case with Alzheimer's disease today. Of course, it was also the only way of discovering an unexpected condition such as a brain tumor or vascular malformation in the brain. It is astonishing to realize that 50 years earlier, the brain of Nietzsche's father had been examined after his death by a country physician while Nietzsche, who was under the care of an eminent researcher in the pathology of general paresis, was allowed to be lowered into his grave without even a simple inspection of his brain.

Besides the intrinsic interest in the neurological aspects of the case itself, Nietzsche had become a world famous personality by the time of his death. Binswanger must have known that there would be great interest generated in the future about the cause of his illness. Neuropathological studies would not only be important to medical science, but to those interested in Nietzsche as a cultural figure. This has been the case, an enormous quantity of ink has been spilled trying to prove one or another view about why Nietzsche suffered a nervous breakdown from which he never recovered. If a postmortem study had been carried out, as was clearly indicated, at least the question of general paresis would have been settled since there are characteristic brain changes in this disease which would have been well-known to any experienced neuropathologist of that era.

The only possible reason for not performing the study would be failure to obtain the consent of the family. However, this appears not to be the case. As stated above, Binswanger was highly regarded by both Frau Nietzsche and Elisabeth, and was sought after many times for his advice. The evidence that the problem was not one of a refusal of consent comes from a letter written by Elisabeth Förster-Nietzsche in 1904, apparently in response to a question about this subject, "Indeed I must confess, that at the time of his death, I never thought about permitting a dissection. No physician had ever made this suggestion . . . besides, at that time the disgusting suspicion [of a syphilitic infection] had not yet emerged."[9]

One of the purposes of a postmortem study is to prove or disprove "suspicions" that may exist in the minds of the family of a deceased person. This was not fulfilled in the case of Friedrich Nietzsche. The specter of syphilis was to haunt his sister throughout her life. Whatever one may think of her character or mentality, she was entitled to know the cause of her brother's death with as much certainty as could be provided by the medical profession. In this respect, Nietzsche's physicians seem to have failed in their responsibility.

A last word needs to be said about certain peculiar references to this question of a postmortem examination. Würzbach, in his annotated selection of Nietzsche's letters, makes a cryptic comment that the sister "hindered" performance of a postmortem study.[10] He gives no reference for this statement. On the other hand, in an ophthalmological article published in 1978, Fuchs offhandedly asserts that "after Nietzsche's death, the diagnosis was histologically confirmed by Ziehen."[11] He also gives no reference for this statement, which seems on the surface to be incredible since nowhere else has any evidence emerged that Ziehen performed such an examination. Möbius, who was familiar with all the circumstances, stated in his monograph that "Unfortunately an autopsy was not performed."[12] This is a subject that bears further study by Nietzsche scholars, if only to preserve the reputation of Nietzsche's psychiatrists.

9

Dementia Paralytica versus Dementia Praecox

DEMENTIA PARALYTICA (GENERAL PARESIS)

The diagnosis of "paresis" (syphilitic brain disease), which was applied to Nietzsche in the year 1889, needs to be evaluated in the context of the understanding of the disease at that time. As previously discussed, the entire field of psychiatry had undergone a radical change in the nineteenth century. The old belief that mentally deranged individuals were somehow in bondage to the devil and had to be kept in chains was replaced by the realization that there was such a thing as mental illness which required intelligence and compassion for its amelioration. It is traditional to credit Philippe Pinel (1745–1826), Professor of Medicine at the University of Paris, with the first effort to free mental patients from their chains and apply enlightened thought to their management.

Pinel divided "insanity" into various categories: melancholia, mania (with or without delirium), dementia, and idiocy. Dementia was characterized by a breakdown in thought processes and, as Redlich and Freedman have suggested, probably consisted of cases of schizophrenia and paresis thrown together.[1] Dementia, that is to say the loss of previously acquired mental abilities, was distinguished from amentia or idiocy which existed from birth.

Later, it was realized that mania and dementia often coexisted in the same individual, manifesting themselves at different times. Pinel's principal approach to treatment was reeducation of the "moral" faculties. While Pinel's treatment theories were later abandoned, his humane approach to mental patients remained an ideal which mental institutions still strive to achieve.

In the early years of the nineteenth century, a number of French physicians—Esquirol, Bayle, Calmeil—made the observations that led to the modern definition of general paresis of the insane, *Paralyse* in German clinical psychiatry. It was noted that a certain number of severely deranged individuals exhibited a general paralysis of their physical capacities which resulted in bodily breakdown and death. Pathological studies of some of these individuals revealed the presence of chronic inflammation of the brain and its covering membranes—meningitis—which suggested that the mental disorder was produced by an underlying brain disease. This was an enormous advance in scientific psychiatry because it was the first clear evidence that mental illness could be produced by a destructive process in the brain. Possession by the devil was clearly out as the explanation of the mental disorder.

It was not long before observations were being made that there was a strikingly high correlation between the presence of a syphilitic infection and the occurrence of the mental disease called general paralysis (*paralysie générale des aliénés*) by Calmeil. However, the mental disease did not occur at the time of the primary syphilitic infection, but rather emerged many years later; five to fifteen years was the usual interval, although periods of up to 30 years were reported. It was this prolonged interval between the acquisition of syphilis and manifestation of mental illness that contributed to the frightening aspect of this disease. No one could know when it might break out, it was actually felt that the less severe cases of syphilis were the ones that were more likely to culminate in a general paralysis. This was the major factor leading to the widespread *syphilophobia* of the nineteenth century. Often overlooked was the fact that only a very small percentage of patients with syphilis went on to develop paralysis, variably estimated at two to four percent. Still, since perhaps up to 10 percent of adult males contracted the disorder at some time, the number of paretics in Europe was thought to be very considerable. Similarities to AIDS (acquired immunodeficiency syndrome) are striking; a sexually transmitted disorder, uniformly lethal, long interval between infection and disease manifestations. Consideration of the fear of AIDS today will give insight into the syphilophobia of nineteenth century.

The final proof of the connection of syphilis to general paresis did not come until 1913 when a Japanese researcher named H. Noguchi, working in the Rockefeller Institute of New York, demonstrated the spirochete of syphilis in a number of brains of individuals with general paresis. This unequivocally established the connection. However, many clinicians did not accept that *all* cases of paresis were due to syphilis. Interestingly enough, one of these holdouts from the doctrine that every case of paresis was due to earlier syphilitic infection was none other than Otto Binswanger, Nietzsche's supervising physician at Jena. Binswanger maintained in an 1894 publication, that some cases of paresis were due to "overexertion" of the brain.[2] This in fact was Elisabeth Förster-Nietzsche's explanation of the cause of her brother's breakdown. One wonders whether his experience with Nietzsche led Binswanger to this point of view. In any case, Binswanger's opinion did not prevail in the scientific community at large, and by the time of Nietzsche's death in 1900, it was generally accepted that paresis was synonymous with syphilitic brain disease. E.H. Hare, in his excellent review of the history of the disorder, suggested that the properties of the spirochete of syphilis changed at about the turn of the eighteenth century to include delayed infection of the brain, which is when general paresis first became widely recognized.[3] This new brain-infecting variant probably was spread throughout Europe by Napoleon's armies. Emigration soon disseminated the disease throughout the world.

The classical description of general paresis was provided by the master clinician Emil Kraepelin in his textbook of psychiatry and in a later monograph by him on the subject.[4] He coined the label *Dementia paralytica* to refer to the disease, a logical diagnostic term because it referred to its two major features, dementia and paralysis. The historical terminology is confusing because writers in different countries have used different expressions. The following all refer to the same condition: progressive paralysis, general paralysis (of the insane), general paresis, paresis, paralysis, dementia paralytica. The term neurosyphilis will also be encountered but this refers to a broader spectrum of diseases than paresis. *General paresis* is the expression usually used in these chapters because it is the most common term used in the English medical literature.

As S.A.K. Wilson put it, in his extensive textbook review prior to the antibiotic era, the symptoms of this disease are almost embarrassing in their profusion.[5] They may mimic any type of functional or organic mental disorder as well as the major psychoses, such as schizophrenia or manic depressive disease. The principal early symptom is usually memory defect along with some alteration of reasoning and critical faculties. These progress to fits of temper, misbehavior, and the development of delusional symptoms. Megalomania was emphasized by early workers but this symptom seemed to be less frequent in the twentieth century. Along with psychiatric abnormalities, there appear abnormal neurological signs, particularly speech disturbances and tremor. Untreated, these inexorably progress to physical helplessness and complete mental deterioration. It was generally agreed that the course of the disease was rapid, lasting from two to four years, with an outside limit of survival of five to six years. In Kraepelin's own series of 244 confirmed cases, 93 percent were dead within five years; the longest survival recorded was eleven years.[6] Sudden onset of an agitated type of paresis, such as Nietzsche might have been thought to exhibit, would often end in demise in a matter of weeks or months, leading to the designation "galloping paralysis."[7] Such cases of paresis were noted well into the twentieth century.[8]

In the nineteenth century, general paresis was regarded as the most dreaded of all causes of insanity because it was the one with the worst outlook. Kraepelin estimated that 10 to 20 percent of all admissions to institutions consisted of paretics, but that figure was much higher if statistics were limited to males. In some institutions, such as the famous Charenton Hospital of Paris, the figure reached almost 50 percent. The institution at Jena had an exceptionally high number of cases of paresis which Binswanger attributed to the fact that many paretics sought cures in the nearby mineral baths of Thuringia.[9] Kraepelin felt that one of the most important responsibilities of the institutional psychiatrist (*Irrenarzt*) was recognition of the presence of general paresis. He made a revealing statement in his influential textbook regarding the diagnosis of paresis: "The common feature of all these disorders [of paretics] is a *characteristic mental weakness* which immediately reveals to the informed examiner the calamitous cause of the entire disease process."[10] It was a matter of professional pride for the institutional physician to be able to recognize paresis among mentally deranged individuals.

In 1913, the advent of the Wasserman test for syphilis forever altered the diagnosis of this disease at all its stages. Diagnosis henceforth was based upon laboratory studies of blood and spinal fluid rather than the psychological and neurological phenomena that had been previously relied on for recognition of the disease. It became evident that paresis had become an overdiagnosed disorder although specific details of the extent of overdiagnosis are hard to come by. Perhaps the most telling disclosure came from Kraepelin himself who confessed that after the availability of laboratory diagnosis, the percentage of paralytics in his clinic fell from 30 percent to 8 to 9 percent![11] This was an astonishing admission from the founder of descriptive clinical psychiatry. Subsequently, the whole emphasis on the diagnosis of general paresis lay on emphasizing the difficulty in distinguishing it from other psychiatric or organic disorders, including schizophrenia and manic depressive psychosis. It became standard to perform one of the serological tests for syphilis on all patients who presented with serious mental disorders because of the difficulties in distinguishing paresis from other psychiatric conditions. This is still the case even though general paresis has virtually disappeared as a clinical entity, at least in the United States and Western Europe.

One of the last major studies of general paresis was conducted in Germany in the 1960s by Wilhelm Zeh and associates.[12] They gave the final *coup de grace* to the idea that paresis could be diagnosed by clinical psychiatric means. The psychiatric manifestations of paralysis are the least significant findings in recognizing this disorder. The diagnosis is essentially a matter of special laboratory studies and specific neurological signs, particularly those involving speech. Without these features, the diagnosis can be nothing more than a hypothesis. "The psychopathological findings possess only limited diagnostic significance. One cannot tell whether they are due to organic brain damage or endogenous factors [schizophrenia, manic depressive disease] or to particular psychological interactions. A specificity of psychopathological symptoms can no longer be entertained today."[13] Other investigators confirmed these findings.[14] The clinical manifestations do not serve to distinguish the disorder from other mental or physical diseases. Only the laboratory findings permit definite diagnosis. Thus scientific medicine moved full circle from the nineteenth century idea that paresis could be diagnosed solely from the appearance and behavior of the patient.

Finally, attention needs to be given to the surprising disappearance of general paresis in the modern world. No single factor suffices to explain this phenomenon. In the beginning of the twentieth century, it was already noted that frequency of the disorder was decreasing. An early authority on paresis, A. Hoche, made this remarkable prediction in 1912: "the younger ones among us will see the day in which paresis will be of only historical interest."[15] Zeh noted that his words have been fulfilled. Hare's review, mentioned above, asserts that when deaths due to dementia paralytica were first recorded in 1901 in England and Wales, they amounted to 2,272. In 1957, they were 68. Today, one may speculate, they are zero. Similar data can be found in most developed countries where such records are maintained. In Kraepelin's classic 1896 *Textbook of Psychiatry*, 80 pages are devoted to dementia paralytica. Today, the disease is usually no more than a single entry in lists of conditions causing organic brain disease. Sometimes a paragraph or two may be given concentrating on historical aspects of the disorder. One would be hard pressed to find a contemporary psychiatrist or neurologist who has ever seen a case of paresis.

The disappearance of the disease is often attributed to the effect of antibiotics but is more likely due to the mutability of the spirochete. Paresis was already showing a marked downturn prior to the antibiotic era. Better diagnosis of mental disorders and prevention of syphilitic infections may have played a role but could not be responsible for the apparent total disappearance of the entity. Syphilis itself has not disappeared, in fact it is increasing; it has been estimated that there are 100,000 new cases per annum in the United States. Some of these must be untreated and could be expected occasionally to develop into paresis. However, such seems not to be the case. There are occasional patients manifesting evidence of syphilis of the central nervous system but virtually never with the full-blown picture of general paresis. Along with St. Vitus' dance, epidemic encephalitis lethargica, and tuberculosis of the brain, general paresis seems to have disappeared from the spectrum of human mental disorders—at least up to the end of the twentieth century.

DEMENTIA PRAECOX (SCHIZOPHRENIA)

In a certain way, schizophrenia may be regarded as the mirror image of general paresis. In the nineteenth century, when general paralysis of the insane was a well-defined entity and considered the most serious problem of mental institutions, schizophrenia was not yet recognized as a clinical entity. Cases that would today be diagnosed as schizophrenic disorder were then described as moral insanity, dementia, mania, catatonia, and so forth. A later survey of the Jena institution, in particular, indicated that one-third of the admissions in 1889 might be diagnosed as schizophrenia, according to current criteria.[16] It was Kraepelin's perceptive clinical insight which resulted in his concept of *dementia praecox*, an acquired thought disorder which took many forms, appeared in early adult life (hence praecox) and almost always resulted in progressive mental deterioration (dementia). By the beginning of the twentieth century, Kraepelin's concept was widely accepted in Western psychiatry. Additionally, Kraepelin distinguished manic depressive insanity, which did *not* invariably result in dementia and began at a later stage of life compared to dementia praecox. Kraepelin's descriptions provided a wealth of detail on dementia praecox, particularly the advanced form of the disease which resulted in a virtually vegetative state for individuals so affected.[17]

Later, psychiatrists began to realize that this disorder did not invariably result in the degree of mental deterioration described by Kraepelin. Treatment was possible and many patients made an adjustment to life without descent into total mental deterioration. While early adulthood is the usual time for onset of schizophrenia, some cases begin later so that the latest version of the American Psychiatric Association's *Manual of Mental Disorders* drops any age requirement for initial diagnosis. Previously, the arbitrary cutoff age had been 45 years. The Swiss psychiatrist Eugen Bleuler de-emphasized the dementia aspect of the disorder when he coined the term "schizophrenia" which has replaced dementia praecox as the accepted descriptive label. Schizophrenia refers to the splitting of psychic functions between fantasy and reality, which is the hallmark of the disease. Like Kraepelin, Bleuler thought schizophrenia to be due to some undiscovered brain disorder. This is still the view of most psychiatrists regarding the origin of schizophrenia. Subsequently, the American psychiatrists Adolph Meyer and Harry Stack Sullivan emphasized the environmental causes of schizophrenia but these are usually thought to be contributory rather than causal factors.

The most important thought disorder in schizophrenia involves delusions, particularly those with a persecutory content. Lehman states "The conviction of being controlled by some unseen mysterious power that exercises its influence from a distance is almost pathognomonic [diagnostic certainty] for schizophrenia."[18] Many other manifestations of thought disorder may be present, resulting in bizarre and incoherent speech that seems to have no basis in reality. Hallucinations, auditory or visual, are common. There is a strong tendency of affected individuals to withdraw their interest from the outside world. Today, schizophrenia is the most common serious mental disorder in the United States and Europe. The majority of non-elderly individuals admitted to mental institutions carry this diagnosis. It is a difficult disorder to manage because of its chronicity and its pervasive effects on the personality, disturbing the fundamental sense of self. The availability of antipsychotic drugs has revolutionized the medical treatment of schizophrenia, resulting in the near disappearance of the totally regressed patient confined to institutional back wards which was the usual outcome of the disorder in Kraepelin's time. However drugs do not cure the disorder. In the twentieth century, recognition of schizophrenic conditions replaced general paresis as the principal preoccupation of psychiatrists who are responsible for severely mentally disordered individuals.

For those who are interested in the cause of Nietzsche's slow regression into a deteriorated mental state, the description of Kraepelin regarding the usual outcome of dementia praecox in the late nineteenth century is worth considering because it closely describes his final condition:

Usually the disease process progresses to deepest imbecility (Blödsinn). The patient withdraws more and more, becomes imbecilic, unresponsive and loses all appreciation of his surroundings. Often he spills or smears his food, dirties himself, holds back feces and urine, salivates on his clothes. All personal initiative is finally extinguished, he remains sitting or standing wherever he may be, mute and lethargic; at most, occasionally laughing to himself in a senseless manner or softly murmuring an occasional meaningless word or phrase; he must then be dressed and undressed, fed, moved about.

Toward external influences, he behaves at times passive and unresponsive, at times resistive. The scant answers which are elicited from him are usually meaningless, and betray only here and there a certain understanding of the question; insistent but simple requests are sometimes obeyed, earlier acquaintances may be correctly named. Here and there appear fragments of earlier schooling, of readings or writings, impressions of historical, geographical or linguistic reminiscences. In the course of time, these remnants of earlier experiences disappear so that finally only an occasional residual reminiscence is evidence that one is dealing, not with an uncultivated or unfruitful field, but a devastated one.[19]

Kraepelin goes on to say much more about the deteriorated condition of individuals with dementia praecox. There are speech disorders: echolalia (repetitions), verbigeration (word salad), klanging, barking, and incoherence. He remarks that there are often neurological signs such as exaggerated reflexes, facial nerve "phenomena," trembling and pupillary differences. Some cases exhibit attacks of total paralysis. He recognized that many cases could be confused with dementia paralytica, particularly when paranoid delusions are present. Here he states that the earlier age of onset in dementia praecox, the lack of memory disturbances and the neurological signs will help in diagnosis. As we have seen, however, there is no absolute clinical distinction between these conditions. It is now known that Kraepelin was wrong on this point; many schizophrenics exhibit major memory impairment relative to other behavior disturbances.[20] Kurt Goldstein, whose studies of the effect of brain damage on language are fundamental to the field, emphasized the similarity of personality deterioration in schizophrenia and organic brain diseases (prior to the antipsychotic drug era). Performance on mental tests showed both groups exhibiting impairment of the capacity for abstract thought. For this reason, Goldstein believed some type of brain dysfunction was at work in schizophrenia.[21]

Unlike paresis, dementia praecox did not usually progress rapidly to death, although the patients with this disorder exhibited a higher mortality than normal individuals. While psychotropic drugs altered the usual downward progression of the disorder, Manfred Bleuler, the son of Eugen Bleuler, estimated in 1941 that one quarter of schizophrenics ultimately deteriorated to a regressed state.[22] There can be little doubt that many cases of slow-moving paresis in the era prior to serological diagnosis, the so-called "stationary" paralysis, would be today diagnosed as schizophrenia.

10

Controversies over Diagnosis

When Nietzsche became famous during the last decade of the nineteenth century, it was only known that he had gone mad, had required care in a mental institution, and was subsequently in seclusion under the care of his family. This provided a certain mystique to his persona and undoubtedly contributed to his fame. Nothing was known by the public about any medical specifics of his mental problems.

The privacy of his medical history was abruptly lost in 1902 with the publication of the previously cited monograph by Paul Möbius titled *On the Pathological in Nietzsche*. In the discussion, Möbius revealed that Nietzsche had suffered with general paresis, a syphilitic disease of the brain which produced insanity and ultimately death in those so affected. The major portion of the monograph analyzed Nietzsche's writings with the purpose of showing how they were affected by his brain disease. This method of literary analysis was known by the name of "pathography," an approach which had been used previously by Möbius and others for the enlightenment of readers. Möbius himself had published pathographic articles about Rousseau, Goethe, Schopenhauer, and Robert Schumann. It is of interest that syphilis is never mentioned in the essay even though Möbius was one of the prominent physicians involved in attribution of paresis to syphilis. This was out of a sense of deference to the sensibilities of the family, that is, Elisabeth Förster-Nietzsche, and the many adherents to Nietzsche's philosophy. It is an interesting commentary on the sexual mores of the time that it was acceptable to attribute a degenerative brain disease to Nietzsche but not a sexually acquired disorder.

Möbius in his essay tells the reader nothing regarding how he came to know that Nietzsche suffered with paresis. It is a pre-established fact; Möbius' interest is in showing how the disease affected his personality and his writings. Since it is a given fact, there could be no discussion as to the merits of the diagnosis or other possible considerations. On page 103, he briefly mentions why his disease could not have been a brain hemorrhage; but, that is the extent of his differential diagnosis. In fact, it is known from other sources how he came upon his information. Möbius was given access to Nietzsche's medical records at Jena with the consent of the sister who apparently had no idea what was in them. There he came upon the diagnosis of paresis that he accepted at face value. He also must have seen the entry about syphilis but chose not to repeat that part of the records for the reasons mentioned above.

Möbius was a facile writer as well as being a prominent neurologist and psychiatrist. He had received a Ph.D. prior to his medical degree. His prose is easily understood by a non-medical reader, which is one reason why his essay was so widely circulated. He was prone, however, to specious generalizations; for example, he starts his essay saying: "The specialist [in mental disorders] cannot doubt at the onset that a man like Nietzsche was affected by a hereditary problem stemming from a family burdened with neurological illnesses . . . If one finds a flower in full bloom, one knows it can not have arisen from wild shrubbery, in the same way, the aberrancies of Nietzsche could not arise from normal people." This was quite unwarranted; Nietzsche's mother and sister, whatever their personality limitations, were "normal people" and his father's brain tumor was generally accepted, even by Möbius, not to represent a hereditary problem. The occasional examples of mental disorder in his extended family do not justify assigning hereditary mental disease to Nietzsche. On page 8, he states that "someone known to me" had told him that Nietzsche's "guardian" in childhood (?) had said he thought Nietzsche would end in a lunatic asylum. These kind of vague statements detract from the value of the essay.

On the Pathological in Nietzsche is an informative writing, even if the author was too glib in many of his assertions. There is much information about the youthful Nietzsche's musical and literary interests, and his personal relationships at Basel. Möbius is particularly informative about Nietzsche's migraine headaches, a disorder with which he himself suffered. He understood how Nietzsche's discontent with his role as a professor of philology led to worsening of his migraine. But basically, Möbius was not sympathetic to Nietzsche's personality. Aside from the question of paralysis which Möbius tactfully referred to as due to an "exogenous" illness originating from a "poison" entering the body, he thought that Nietzsche's personality exhibited, from the beginning, signs of "degeneration" (*Entartung*), a theory about *fin-de-siècle* "free spirits" that had been elaborated by Max Nordau[1] and later reached its culmination in National Socialist doctrine. His final statement at the end of the essay has been widely quoted and may be viewed as a curse which Möbius pronounced upon Nietzsche and has remained with him to this day:

People read Nietzsche's writings but they don't evaluate them so as to retain the best, rather they fixate on certain ones with which they agree and assume that all the rest are well-founded. Their trust is supported by certain literary men and women who idealize the great philosopher and assure the public that his pearls all hang together on an invisible connecting braid. Who is capable of an independent judgment? Perhaps one among a hundred readers. To those other ninety-nine one must say: If you find pearls, don't think that they all are genuine. Be suspicious, because this man has a sickness of the brain.

It did not take long for the implication of the diagnosis of paresis to be realized by those interested in Nietzsche. He must have acquired syphilis at an earlier age if general paresis was the cause of his mental derangement. It was soon learned that the diagnosis of syphilis was explicitly mentioned in the Jena records. The Basel records only indicate that the patient "indicated that he infected himself twice," a frequent euphemism, however, for referring to syphilitic infection. Elisabeth was outraged at the diagnosis, she had always considered her brother to be a model of chastity; syphilis did not fit into her effort to create an image of him as a spiritual pioneer of German intellectual life. She marshaled his former friends and colleagues to dispute the allegation. As mentioned in an earlier chapter, Nietzsche was a person who was thought to have no interest in the physical aspects of his relationships with women and was thought likely to have been celibate his entire life. In fact, this was untrue as indicated by Dr. Otto Eiser's reports, as well as the evidence from the Jena and Basel records that he demanded women during his manic periods and had delusions of whores in his room. However, this information was not publicly available at the time of the controversy.

The question arose as to who told Nietzsche's physicians that there had been a syphilitic infection. Initially, suspicion was centered on Franz Overbeck as the possible culprit because he was the one who had delivered Nietzsche to the Basel institution and had had conferences with Binswanger about Nietzsche. It would have been impossible to believe that Frau Nietzsche, the other major informant, could have said such a thing about her son. Overbeck indignantly denied the accusation; it was so upsetting to him that the episode was thought to have contributed to his death from heart disease shortly afterwards. Finally, however, Professor Binswanger admitted that there was no record in the chart indicating the source of the information. Presumably it came from the patient's own statement at Friedmatt, a very unreliable source considering Nietzsche's mental state at the time. Perhaps Nietzsche was referring to the gonorrhea—*Tripper*—which he had admitted to Eiser. However, all these disputes were irrelevant once it was accepted that Nietzsche's mental condition was due to paresis. The cause of general paresis, according to modern medicine, is syphilis whether or not a history of a primary infection is available.

In order to put into perspective much of the controversy about syphilis and Nietzsche, it is necessary to have an understanding of the natural course of the disease in humans as scientists have come to understand it over the past two centuries. The initial manifestations of syphilis affect the genitals, producing the lesion known as a chancre; other parts of the body may be affected later (secondary syphilis) during the first one to two years of the disease. Secondary syphilis represents the spreading of the spirochete

(*Treponema pallidum*) throughout the organism. The symptoms may be very varied which gave rise to the famous phrase attributed to Sir Jonathan Hutchinson that syphilis was "the great imitator." However, the disease is not life-threatening in these early stages and almost always spontaneously resolves without leaving traces.

The problem with syphilis is that the spirochete may not completely leave the body and may produce symptoms many years after the primary infection. This is the so-called tertiary phase of syphilis which may affect various organs including the heart, the skin, the bones and, the most dreaded of all late effects, the brain and spinal cord. Exactly how and why these late manifestations occur is still a mystery, quite analogous to the mystery of why AIDS occurs so long after HIV infection. However, unlike the almost invariable appearance of AIDS some time after HIV infection, the tertiary manifestations of syphilis only occur in a minority of patients who have exhibited the primary infection. General paresis has always been a relatively infrequent complication of syphilitic infection. Even in the heyday of the disorder, Kraepelin estimated that no more than 4.75 percent of patients with syphilis developed this disorder.[2] In the twentieth century, even this small figure steadily diminished until the present time when it must be regarded as a medical rarity.

These figures mean that it is largely irrelevant as to whether Nietzsche contracted primary syphilis. It would be a minor detail of his personal life. Since only one in 25 or one in 50 individuals with syphilis went on to manifest general paresis, the prior occurrence of syphilis in an individual manifesting a psychotic breakdown is hardly convincing evidence that it must represent general paresis. Conversely, it was noted that many cases of serologically proven paresis gave no history of prior syphilis which was explained on the belief that it was the milder cases of syphilis that gave rise to the more serious tertiary manifestations. The point is that the diagnosis of general paresis must be made independently and not because a history of syphilis is elicited prior to the disease manifestations under consideration. The meaningful question with respect to Nietzsche's position in European culture is whether he was a victim of general paresis or whether his mental breakdown should be attributed to his intrinsic psychic structure irrespective of the clinical psychiatric diagnosis which may be attached to it. The question is whether the curse of Möbius was well founded—was Nietzsche suffering with a disease of his brain?—not whether he had contracted a case of syphilis in his youth.

A more medically valid analysis of Nietzsche's illness was published in 1925 by Kurt Hildebrandt, entitled *Health and Illness in Nietzsche's Life and Work*. Hildebrandt was a psychiatrist who was chief physician at a Berlin psychiatric clinic. He also was recipient of a Ph.D. in philosophy and had previously published papers on Nietzsche's philosophical positions. By this time, Nietzsche's position in the world of German culture was well-established; Hildebrandt was an important admirer who wished to protect his reputation from Möbius' implication that his work was tainted by brain disease. But he was also a perceptive psychiatrist whose analysis of Nietzsche's illness still stands as one of the best works on the subject.

Hildebrandt recognized that Nietzsche's migraine headaches and myopic eyestrain were influenced by his life's circumstances, that is, were strongly psychosomatic in nature. He produced many objections to the belief that Nietzsche had contracted syphilis. More importantly, he mentioned the reasons for suspecting the validity of the diagnosis of general paresis: The lack of characteristic speech or handwriting findings, the long duration of the illness, and the absence of intellectual deficit prior to onset of the psychosis. Hildebrandt did not have available to him the records of the Jena institutionalization, which had mysteriously disappeared from the files. However, he was in correspondence with both Binswanger and Ziehen who provided him with the relevant information about Nietzsche's condition in Jena. He quotes Ziehen as saying with respect to other possibilities: "Schizophrenia is not a consideration if one understands this term in the broader sense of many German psychiatrists. . . ." Regarding schizophrenia, Hildebrandt views it as a plausible diagnosis. However, he rejects it because "the diagnosis would thereby only be more complicated because one must also assume the presence of a frank organic brain disorder."[3] He finally states that "I believe, therefore, that we should be content with the diagnosis of 'paresis' [or cerebral lues]. Nonetheless, other diagnoses may well have merit since we must remember that the diagnosis of a syphilitic infection cannot be regarded as proven."[4] Apparently Hildebrandt felt that the last stage of Nietzsche's illness necessitated the diagnosis of some form of organic brain disease. However he is not explicit on this point.

In 1930, a German philologist named Erich Podach created a sensation in the world of Nietzsche commentary by publishing the heretofore missing records of Nietzsche's care in the Jena institution.[5] He had apparently obtained the copy from a German periodical (*Der National Zeitung*). By a strange twist of fate, the original records appeared shortly after, having been discovered in the lodgings of a former assistant physician at Jena. Podach was criticized greatly for this daring act as engaging in unauthorized and incompetent lay interference in medical jurisdiction, although he had deleted some of what he felt to be objectionable material in the records. Later, the complete record was published by Verrechia, Volz, and others. Podach was not shy, in spite of his lay status, in pointing out the uncertainties of the diagnosis of general paresis. He circulated Nietzsche's records to experts of his own choosing who were decidedly mixed in their opinions about Nietzsche's diagnosis.[6] Most of them referred to the uncertainties of diagnosis without significant neurological findings and without laboratory data. The scantiness of the recordkeeping was emphasized. A Dr. Michaelis said that the peculiar psychomotor behavior was suggestive of a schizophrenic psychosis. Dr. Stutz, chief physician of the Basel clinic, felt that while the diagnosis of the Basel clinic (40 years earlier) was uncertain, the records at Jena confirmed the diagnosis of progressive paralysis. He went on to say that he regarded Nietzsche as a "schizoid" personality who died from syphilitic brain disease. It is of interest that Dr. Stutz went on to add that he found in the Basel records of that era many cases of paresis which today would be definitely regarded as schizophrenia.

Karl Jaspers is one of the principal figures of twentieth century philosophy whose life and productivity rival that of Nietzsche's in interest. He is one of the band of philosopher-psychiatrists who are known as *Nietzsche-Kenner*—connoisseurs of Nietzsche (Möbius, Ziehen, Hildebrandt, Lange-Eichbaum, Benda). Jaspers is the most famous of them all; his name will always be associated with the German existentialist movement in philosophy. Jaspers began his career in psychiatry, producing for 30 years his classic textbook titled *General Psychopathology* whose last edition appeared in 1946.

During the Nazi era, Jaspers was dismissed from his post as professor of philosophy at Heidelberg because of his Jewish wife. They were prevented from emigrating; his wife had to go into hiding to escape the Gestapo. Finally they were both scheduled for transportation to concentration camps, which Jaspers only avoided through American occupation of Heidelberg. After the war, he accepted an appointment at the University of Basel where he remained until his death in 1969.

Because of his background, Jaspers' book titled *Nietzsche*, which first appeared in 1936 in Nazi Germany, is of particular interest. The principal focus of the book is Nietzsche's philosophical positions which Jaspers handles in highly thoughtful, if somewhat ambiguous manner. However, the first part deals with Jaspers' views on Nietzsche's life and illnesses. He is quite circumspect in labeling Nietzsche's illness. He enigmatically refers to a "biological factor" which he thinks was operative in Nietzsche's life from the mid-1880s. There is no doubt, however, that he considers this "factor" to be probably syphilis of the brain.[7] He categorically states that "the mental illness at the end of 1888 is an organic brain disease which derives from an external cause and not from an inner disposition."[8] Regarding schizophrenia, he states, "To designate the process as schizophrenia or as schizoid seems futile to me, since such diagnostic categories are, at their very best, ill-defined and etiologically meaningless."[9] All this is very similar to the views expressed by Hildebrandt in his monograph. There is a certain hesitancy in Jaspers' discussions of Nietzsche's illness which is characteristic of the book in general. It is sometimes difficult to know exactly what Jaspers means. One must remember the circumstances under which the book was written and the fact that Nietzsche, at least initially, was in the Nazi pantheon of heroes. Jaspers clearly alludes to this in his preface to later reprints of the book.

Following the Second World War, Nietzsche fell into general disrepute as he was considered part of the catastrophic political movement which had plunged the world into so much war and misery. It was felt to be quite appropriate that the philosophical source of the *Übermensch* doctrine should be a syphilitic whose brain had been devoured by spirochetes. This point of view survives to the present day. However in 1965, a German psychiatrist named Kurt Kolle produced a paper with a new idea about Nietz-

sche's illness.[10] The article quotes Jaspers' descriptions of Nietzsche's behaviors at great length to which he appends the following
noteworthy statement:

A modern psychiatrist, who reads this medical history of the 35–46 year
old Nietzsche, who does not know that it deals with Nietzsche, would
hardly hesitate to declare; *here is visible the classical features of manic-
depressive (cyclothymic) phases.*

Verrechia also stated that his psychiatric consultant felt Nietzsche's problem was manic-depressive psychosis.[11] The exact quote
of the unnamed consultant was "What does 'progressive paralysis' mean! Manic psychosis; that was Nietzsche's illness!" In the
1970s, when Verrecchia was canvassing psychiatrists about Nietzsche's breakdown, general paresis was already virtually an extinct
concept.

Nevertheless, Kolle does not completely discard the possibility of
general paresis. He felt that the views of experienced psychiatrists
like Wille, Binswanger, and Ziehen could not be ignored; he attributed the final stages of Nietzsche's illness to organic brain disease.
His position was that the "cyclothymic undulations may have pre-
cipitated the organic process." Here he reverses the explanation of
others who believed that paresis could precipitate an endogenous
psychosis, that is, schizophrenia or a manic-depressive disorder. It
is curious that Kolle feels Hildebrandt, Jaspers, and Benda may
have not had sufficient experience with manic-depressive disease
to recognize its features.

No review of the opinions about Nietzsche's illness could be
complete without consideration of the writings of Clemens Benda
on the subject. Elderly neurologists may be familiar with the name
of Clemens Benda as the author of one of the first works in child
neurology titled *Developmental Disorders of Mentation and Cerebral
Palsies* published in 1952. It was a landmark publication and still
contains some of the most comprehensive descriptions of the neuropathology of brain-damaged children. Those who know the
name of Benda will be surprised (as was this writer) to learn that
he was also an authority on the life and illness of Friedrich Nietzsche. Benda describes himself as a young psychiatrist attending
Karl Jaspers' philosophical seminars in Heidelberg when he was
commissioned by Jaspers to obtain material about Nietzsche's life

and illness. As part of the investigation, he had the opportunity to hold many conversations with Otto Binswanger who, although retired, still had a vivid memory of Nietzsche. Benda published his materials in 1925 where he takes the position that general paresis was the most likely explanation of Nietzsche's illness.[12] Schizophrenia is discarded because of the rapidity of onset of the psychosis. The diagnosis of migraine is discarded because Benda thinks Nietzsche's headaches were due to syphilitic meningitis. Chronic chloral hydrate use may have contributed to Nietzsche's sudden breakdown as was originally believed by Binswanger.

Benda must have subsequently emigrated to the United States since he was director of research at the Fernald State School in Massachusetts during the 1940s and 1950s. In 1965, he again entered into the fray of Nietzsche diagnosis with a two-part article titled "On the Illness of Friedrich Nietzsche."[13] Most of the content deals with Nietzsche's life and writings with which Benda is most empathetic and admiring. However, at the end, he returns to the question of diagnosis. His opinions of 40 years have not changed one iota. He is the authoritative expert professional who brooks no objection to his opinions. It is worth quoting Benda at length because his views best represent the professional judgments that led to the diagnosis of syphilitic brain disease in Nietzsche:

Concerning the diagnosis, both clinics, Basel and Jena, established it as general paresis. Although at that time, neither the Wassermann-reaction nor examination of the spinal fluid was available, the clinical picture of general paresis had been worked out so well that the discovery of serological reactions was only a helpful confirmation of the diagnosis. The clinical picture had already been so completely observed and described before the Wassermann epoch that later researchers could only add some finer details.

Actually, no psychiatric specialist who learned his psychiatry before 1930 when experiences with syphilis and paresis occurred daily in major clinics has doubted the diagnosis in Nietzsche's case. All the criticisms have come from lay people, even some medical ones, whose remarks are better passed over in sil nce. I don't think it necessary to discuss the long closed records in detail: in the entire history of medicine there is no other illness, in spite of all the many new infectious disorders that have been discovered in our century, in which such a unique combination of neurological symptoms and specific mental disturbances are present. The frightening aura of megalomania, irritability, agitation alternating with placidity, flight of ideas and incoherence of thought and speech, aggressiveness and self-depreciation, smearing of feces, drinking urine, lalling speech, facial paralysis, unequal pupils and tremor, all these phenomena were observed in Nietzsche. No schizophrenic lives in so many different worlds at the same time, no other illness has such a frightful spectrum of breakdown from which there is no return. A quicksilver [mercury] cure apparently checked the intensity of the symptoms and arrested their rapid progress. On March 24, 1890, Nietzsche was discharged after a 14-month stay. He lived ten years, being reduced to the level of a helpless child. Paralysis, speech disturbances and other neurological symptoms reduced the physical state of this once strong and well-built man to a shade of his earlier self.

Benda writes with a vivid style and a strong sense of self-assurance. However, objections must be raised to some of his assertions. It is simply not true that psychiatric specialists trained before 1930 had no doubt about the diagnosis of progressive paralysis in Nietzsche. Kurt Hildebrandt whose description and analysis of Nietzsche's illness is still the best available had grave doubts about the diagnosis, which he finally accepted as the most reasonable supposition. Podach's consultants previously quoted had mixed views about its correctness. In fact, the entire direction of thoughts about diagnosis of general paresis from the 1920s on was to question its validity without corroborating serological evidence. It became known that diagnoses were often changed following introduction of the Wassermann test; the previously cited experience of Kraepelin, the outstanding authority in this disorder, is only one example of this phenomenon. Wilson's comprehensive textbook discussion prior to introduction of antibiotics asserts the following: "No one mental symptom or syndrome is specific for neurosyphilis, not even the grandiose delusions observed in one half of all cases of general paresis. From the mildest emotional or intellectual trouble to the most profound dementia, to mania, delirious or paranoid state, each and all can be matched in other conditions from which syphilis as a causal agent can be excluded."[14] The monograph of Merritt, Adams, and Solomon on neurosyphilis that sums up the experiences of the pre-antibiotic era states: "Dementia paralytica may be accompanied by symptoms that cannot be differentiated at first sight from those of manic depressive psychosis . . . examination of the cerebrospinal fluid is paramount in diagnosis . . . the preceding statements concerning manic depressive psychosis and dementia paralytica hold also for schizophrenic psychosis."[15]

Zeh, whose assessment of the specificity of the psychopathological features in general paresis has been discussed in Chapter 9, also addresses the question of how "experienced" clinicians recognize the picture of paralysis. This is a similar issue to that of recognition of schizophrenia in which a "praecox feeling" has been described which requires personal contact of an experienced psychiatrist with the patient. Zeh concludes that a similar "paresis feeling" is not based on the psychiatric picture alone but requires certain neurological abnormalities, specifically speech disturbances [articulation], slack facial features, widespread tremors, movement disorders, and psychomotor decline. "What is thought to be typical of paresis is in reality a *complex somatic and psychic ensemble of symptoms* which indicates extensive cerebral damage including frontal and temporal regions. Paresis-like clinical syndromes have been described with brain tumors, atrophic processes, encephalitides and brain injuries."[16] Moreover, regarding Nietzsche's illness, none of the neurological signs and symptoms enumerated by Zeh were reliably described during Nietzsche's period of institutionalization.

Finally, Benda has no basis for saying that the "quicksilver" or mercury cure arrested the progress of Nietzsche's symptoms. Mercury was used in the treatment of primary syphilis with some effectiveness, although the toxicity of effective doses was a serious problem that led to its abandonment when other treatments became available. Most authorities, however, agreed with Wilson who stated that its use in general paresis, a tertiary form of syphilis, was notoriously inadequate.[17] Spontaneous remission of symptoms in endogenous psychosis—manic-depressive or schizophrenic—is common following institutionalization; similar remissions occurred with general paresis but were usually short-lived.

An opposite view of Nietzsche's illness was provided in 1982 in a work titled *Nietzsche, Psychologist of the Depths* by Louis Corman, a French psychiatrist who was interested in Nietzsche's psychological theories. The work is principally devoted to an explanation of Nietzsche's own unique attitudes to the human condition. However, in a note at the end of his monograph, he discusses the question of Nietzsche's madness.[18] Corman states his own experience included several years studying patients with general paresis. He makes the relevant observation that the delusional megalomania which led Nietzsche's physicians to diagnose paresis is a valid indicator of the disease only in the context of dementia, in other words when there are severe deficits of memory and understanding. *Ecce Homo*, written just before the outbreak of his madness, displays a lucid and vigorous thought content and is composed with Nietzsche's usual masterful prose style. There is no evidence in it, according to Corman, of weakening of Nietzsche's mental abilities. Moreover, he points out the absence of dysarthria which is the most characteristic neurological sign of paralysis. He concludes his discussion as follows:

My conclusion is that Nietzsche—in whom a syphilitic infection was, I repeat, more than doubtful—did not suffer with general paresis, but with a *schizophrenic psychosis*, this non-dementing disorder that is the manifestation of an existential break with reality, of a total introversion with his thought blocked and withdrawn into his interior being, with loss of any possibility for external expression.

Exception might be taken to Corman referring to schizophrenia—dementia praecox—as a "non-dementing" disease but his overall analysis is quite to the point. Could the author of *Ecce Homo* have been suffering with syphilitic damage to the brain that in a few weeks would produce total breakdown of Nietzsche's personality? This question will be taken up in more detail in Chapter 12.

The last work of consequence is the comprehensive documentation of Nietzsche's illnesses titled *Nietzsche in the Labyrinth of his Illness* by Pia Daniela Volz. It is a unique publication in that it provides documentation of virtually all the relevant materials concerning Nietzsche's illnesses. This makes it an invaluable source of information for anyone interested in this subject, especially those who cannot journey to Weimar to gain access to the original sources. Volz is very thorough in her inclusion of virtually all relevant information. In the penultimate chapter titled "Looking Back on the History of an Illness," she provides her own opinion about the cause of Nietzsche's illness:

On the 25th of August, 1900 Friedrich Nietzsche died at the age of 55 years in the endstage of a dementia into which he slipped during the last period of life, "helpless as a corpse, in life already dead and buried." The progressive loss of all physical and mental abilities in the course of eleven years corresponds to the picture of an organic brain syndrome. The global destruction of all higher cerebral functions is best explained, in my opinion, by the diagnosis made during his stay at the Basel psychiatric clinic, namely by general paresis, which—as was not known with certainty at that time—is in every case the direct consequence of a syphilitic infection. Other diagnostic hypotheses such as dementia secondary to a stroke, schizophrenia, epilepsy, Borrelia infection (Lyme disease) or medication misuse inferred from the documents cited are not, or only in part, compatible with the symptoms.[19]

It should be noted that Volz bases her opinion upon the deterioration exhibited by Nietzsche during his care by the family, not on the symptoms presented during his stay at the two institutions, Basel and Jena. In essence, she feels that the regression which he demonstrated was indicative of the correctness of the diagnosis of general paresis. The emphasis switches from expert clinicians who know how to recognize general paresis to the reliance upon the presence of total and wide-ranging regression as evidence of the disease. However, the clinical picture of regression is a frail reed upon which to base so specific a diagnosis.[20]

"Six-Seventh Blind"

Among the various physical problems that plagued Nietzsche, the problem of his vision deserves special attention. It was the problem which most interfered with his professional career, giving him a valid excuse for resigning his professorship. He visited more ophthalmologists than any other type of specialist. His loss of vision, as well as the predictions of the ophthalmologists, led him to fear blindness throughout much of his adult life and he often referred to himself in his letters as anywhere between one-half to six-seventh blind. The inflammatory changes described in the interior layers of his eyes were the only objective evidence of significant physical disease observed in Nietzsche during his long years of suffering with eyestrain, headaches, vomiting, back pains, insomnia, hemorrhoids, and general nervous prostration. The question of the origin of this inflammation, otherwise known as chorioretinitis, has been a minor chord in the ensemble of problems dominated by his mental disorder.

His nearsightedness (myopia) and unequal pupils, first noted when he was four years old, have been previously described. Fuchs, whose paper on Nietzsche's eye disorders has been previously mentioned, refers to the "staring" expression seen in his photographs, presumably indicative of severe myopia.[1] The problem began to be really troublesome when he was a schoolboy at

Pforta when it was thought to be the cause of his headaches. This was the beginning of the long-standing uncertainty in the minds of Nietzsche's physicians and in his own mind as to whether his headaches were secondary to his eyestrain or stemmed from primary sources in his head—migraine or otherwise. This problem was never resolved in his lifetime; it is most likely that both mechanisms were operative because there is compelling evidence that Nietzsche also suffered with migraine.

In any case, the degree of myopia measured by the ophthalmologists was quite substantial. As a teenager, the degree of myopia was measured as minus six diopters;[2] by the time he was in Basel, it was said to be between minus thirteen and minus twenty diopters, a problem which was bound to produce eyestrain without adequate correction. The prescription of corrective lenses did not seem to resolve Nietzsche's symptoms, possibly because of the presence of an unrecognized astigmatism. Atropine treatments were recommended in order to rest the muscles of accommodation. Other therapies tried in Basel were eye douches, local bloodletting with leeches, and electrogalvanization. None of these provided any significant relief. Additionally, there was evidence of weakness of the external ocular muscles (strabismus) leading to intermittent double vision. Volz provides many details from the records of his ophthalmologists for those who can decipher German ophthalmological terminology from the nineteenth century.[3] The main point is that Nietzsche was seriously handicapped in the use of his eyes for sustained close work.

There was no evidence of serious problems with his eyes during Nietzsche's period as a university student. Visual problems emerged in full force only when he assumed the professorship at Basel. In retrospect, his decision to take on a career in academic philology was a catastrophic error, not only because his own interests were not in the minutiae of scholarly work but also because his eyes were not up to what was required. In *Ecce Homo*, Why I Am So Wise, *s*.7, he states, no doubt drawing from his own experience: "The scholar who basically only 'leafs' through books—a philologist averages about 200 a day—finally completely loses his ability to think for himself." Elsewhere, he has stated that he could not read for more than twenty minutes without feeling pain.

His visits beginning in 1873 to Professor Schiess, a Basel ophthalmologist, revealed something more besides simple eyestrain, namely, the presence of an inflammation in his retina. Subsequently, all ophthalmologists who examined Nietzsche found changes indicative of chronic inflammation. This was undoubtedly responsible for much of the fluctuations in Nietzsche's symptoms, particularly the sudden changes in vision and the bizarre visual imagery noted when his eyes were closed which led him to wonder if he was becoming insane.[4] The question naturally arises as to the cause of this inflammation in the interior layers of the eyes.

Every textbook dealing with diseases of the eye has long lists of conditions that may produce chorioretinitis—inflammation of inner layers of the eye. Among these are various viral infections, autoimmune disorders, tuberculosis, sarcoidosis, toxoplasmosis, kidney disease, and, of course, syphilis. Today, the obscure disease of toxoplasmosis is believed to be the principal cause of chorioretinitis. However, in practice, the origin of chorioretinitis is rarely established and treatment is based on local measures designed to reduce inflammation and deal with its consequences. It is likely the same was true in the nineteenth century. Prior to his psychotic breakdown, Nietzsche's ophthalmologists did not consider syphilis to be the cause of his chorioretinitis. Dr. Eiser, in the report described in Chapter 4, specifically excluded it as the cause of his eye problems.[5] Yet it is common to find references indicating that Nietzsche's chorioretinitis was a manifestation of his syphilis.

Besides the above-mentioned conditions, it is known that pathologic myopia in time damages the choroid layer of the inner eye and the adjacent retina that is responsible for visual images. This condition is one of the leading causes of blindness today.[6] Initially there occurs thinning and atrophy of the choroid layer resulting in extreme light sensitivity.[7] The retina exhibits hemorrhages, scarring, and degeneration. It is the retinal degeneration, especially in the central macular area most important for vision, which ultimately may produce blindness. Paralysis of pupillary muscles with light unresponsive pupils—one of the signs which suggested syphilis to Nietzsche's physicians—is also a byproduct. The simplest explanation of Nietzsche's chorioretinitis is that it followed upon the severe myopia that plagued him throughout his life. However, there can be no certainty on this point.

In 1878, on the advice of his friend Rohde, Nietzsche went to

Halle for a consultation with Dr. Alfred Graefe, a well-known specialist in diseases of the eye. On the basis of his examination (which was not preserved), Dr. Graefe recommended that Nietzsche give up his professorship and abstain from reading or writing for a period of five years.[8] Supposedly he commented that Nietzsche was an example of the extent to which German scholars can ruin their eyes. Graefe's consultation was the final precipitating factor in Nietzsche's giving up his post as professor of philology.

Perhaps it is best to let Nietzsche himself have the last word on this subject. In a letter to Georg Brandes dated March 27, 1888, he makes the following observation:

I may mention in passing that my eyes are the barometer of my general condition; after fluctuations, they have entered on a period of general improvement, and have become more sound and lasting than I could ever have believed possible. Indeed they have falsified the prophecies of the very best German oculists. If Graefe, the celebrated specialist, *et hoc genus omne*, had been right, I should have been blind long ago. It is bad enough to have come to No. 3 spectacles, but I can still see.

12

What Caused Nietzsche's Breakdown?

In the foreword to *Ecce Homo* composed shortly before the breakdown, Nietzsche wrote: *"Listen to me! I am such and such. Above all, do not be mistaken about me!"* However, Nietzsche has made it very difficult not to be mistaken about him because he has put so many barriers in the way of recognizing who he was. He takes pride in saying throughout his writings that he does not communicate his ideas directly, does not stay with his subject, engages in outrageous hyperbole, is fascinated with the idea of masks and madness, and refuses to express himself plainly about his beliefs. He is far more of a critic than a philosopher, more a moralist—in his own way—than a "psychologist." He makes much of his idea that sickness is necessary for health; yet it is very difficult to pin down the cause of the many ailments that plagued him throughout his life. He often drops hints about the fragility of his own physical constitution but nothing prepares us for the permanent mental collapse which occurred shortly after a period of unparalleled literary creativity. The huge quantity of writings he left behind—the works published by himself, the posthumous publications, his vast correspondence, his notebooks which have been preserved and published, and the many experiences and observations made about him by his friends, family, and physicians greatly complicate the problem of recognizing who he was. Finally, it did not help that his sister, who inherited his literary estate, spent decades creating an image of Nietzsche that had little correspondence with reality.

It is impossible that the cause of his breakdown will ever be established with certainty. There were no confirmatory laboratory procedures which today would be required to establish the diagnosis of general paresis. It is necessary to weigh the probabilities—to consider his behavior, physical symptoms, the opinions of his physicians, the course of his mental illness, and, above all, what is known about the specific conditions from which he might have suffered. Regarding this latter subject, one is in a condition that might be compared to an archaeological investigation. The medical conditions to be considered do not currently exist. General paresis, particularly the so-called classical megalomaniac type, is an extinct disorder, having gone the way of St. Vitus dance and epidemic encephalitis. There is no current experience, one is required to study the musty volumes of a long gone medical milieu. The same is true with respect to the endstage demented schizophrenic although, perhaps, occasional examples of this unfortunate situation might still be found. However, the antipsychotic drugs have dramatically altered the course of schizophrenic disorders leading to avoidance of institutionalization. Kraepelin could not have conceived of caring for most individuals with dementia praecox outside of mental hospitals.

Consideration of Nietzsche's protracted but permanent mental disorder can be divided into four stages reflecting the different circumstances under which it manifested itself. These are the following: (1) onset of psychosis in Turin; (2) mental breakdown with psychiatric evaluations; (3) institutionalization at Jena; and (4) home care in Naumburg and Weimar. His symptoms were different during these periods; these differences cannot automatically be attributed to the progress of his disorder.

1. October–December 1888 (onset of psychosis)

- euphoria and grandiosity
- gradual loss of reality testing
- coherent writing with memory, abstract thinking, and organization intact
- prolonged grimacing
- behavioral aberrations

2. First two weeks of January 1889 (mental breakdown)

- "mad" letters
- manic behavior and flight of ideas
- extreme restlessness
- delusions of grandeur
- psychotic splitting of thought
- absence of neurological abnormalities or intellectual impairment

As Kurt Kolle pointed out in his 1965 publication, Nietzsche's symptoms by this time were highly suggestive of manic-depressive psychosis. The age of onset, the predominance of abnormality of mood, the history of depression and the fact that Nietzsche's bizarre thoughts were congruent with his earlier well worked-out philosophy, pointed away from the diagnosis of a schizophrenic disorder. There were virtually no indications of organic disease other than the pupillary findings which, given his chorioretinitis, could be discounted as an index of organicity. As far as the diagnosis of general paresis is concerned, it can only be explained on the basis of the belief of Nietzsche's psychiatrists that his psychopathology indicated this condition, an assumption that subsequent medical research has shown not to be justified.

3. Late January 1889–March 1890 (institutional care)

- increasing delusions of persecution
- alternation between fantasy and reality in conversation
- hallucinations
- smearing of stool, drinking of urine
- odd behavior; collects scraps and papers
- detailed recollection of past events
- remembers recent conversations and readings
- fearful of strangers
- childishly docile behavior
- plays expressively on piano
- physically healthy
- no significant neurological abnormalities

Nietzsche's condition in the Jena institution gradually changed from one of severe manic disorder to a pervasive thought disorder. The signs and symptoms became more suggestive of a schizophrenic disorder. The remission mentioned in the Jena record of October 1, 1890, referred only to his behavior, his thought disorder was worsening. In the days when psychotic individuals were routinely admitted to mental institutions, it was not uncommon to find a change of diagnosis after a period of time from manic-depressive psychosis to schizophrenia.[1] Another way psychiatrists have found to deal with the difficulty that exists at times in distinguishing between the two major forms of endogenous psychosis is to use the term "schizoaffective disorder."[2] It is not necessary to enter into the complexities of psychiatric terminology to realize that Nietzsche's principal problem at the time was the disorganized and fantastic content of his thought leading to a loss of contact with reality. The manifestation of such a style of thought over a prolonged time period usually leads to a diagnosis of schizophrenia. There were still no obvious neurological abnormalities to suggest an organic brain disease.

4. March 1890–August 1900 (home care at Naumburg, Weimar)

- continuation of thought disorder
- increasing apathy
- loss of volitional activity
- diminishment of speech
- often tired
- easily agitated
- echolalia (repetition of words)
- incoherence of speech
- responsive to music
- confinement to wheel chair
- "automaton-like" behavior
- appearance of "paralytic attacks"

Nietzsche's gradual decay into a vegetative state accompanied by what his sister called "attacks of paralysis" is the principal reason that the diagnosis of general paresis has retained plausibility up to the present time. Attacks of paralysis, strokes as they are called today, were often described in individuals with general paresis. In this day of successful treatment of mental illness, it is difficult to conceive of Nietzsche's deterioration as not being caused by an external factor, specifically, syphilitic brain disease, since that was the diagnosis of his physicians before Nietzsche became "a living corpse." However, this apparently plausible conclusion requires some analysis.

The German word *"Lähmung"* or paralysis had a broader meaning in the late nineteenth century than it does at the present time. It could refer to anything from prostration to true paralysis such as one understands the term today. Nietzsche himself referred in his January 1880 letter to Dr. Eiser to a *"Lähmung"* accompanying his headaches at the time. Binswanger kept on asking Frau Nietzsche about the occurrences of paralysis during her care for him but there were apparently no such events until 1897, long after Nietzsche had sunk into incommunicability. In March 1895, his mother was still saying that he walks with a "forceful stride."[3]

On December 31, 1896, Frau Nietzsche reported periods of weakness which Binswanger thought to finally represent "paralysis" although he was still able to walk about.[4] After their mother's death in 1897, Elisabeth Förster-Nietzsche assumed responsibility for Nietzsche's care. In her later descriptions of her brother's illness, there occur references to a long standing paralysis (right-sided) which supposedly interfered with his speech and gait.[5] Lesser attacks are mentioned and then, in 1899, a more severe attack of paralysis is said to have occurred. She witnessed his death on August 25, 1900, which was associated with fever and signs of congestion of the lungs—probably pneumonia. Elisabeth took the final opportunity to mention an "attack" which occurred some hours before his demise.

None of the observers who provided accounts of Nietzsche's appearance during his last years reported any evidence of a hemiplegia or other signs of sequelae of a stroke. All agreed on his general debility but none mentioned one-sided paralysis. Schumacher mentions *both* hands laying on his blanket; Jesinghaus describes a feeble *right* hand held out in greeting, only a month or so after an "attack" which left him unable to speak according to the sister.[6] Dr. Vulpius who examined his eyes in November 1899 mentions his healthy general appearance and makes no mention of hemiplegia or paralysis.[7,8] One needs to remember that Elisabeth wanted the world to believe Nietzsche was afflicted with strokes. This, along with the after-effects of drug misuse, was her explanation of the cause of Nietzsche's illness. Most scholars of the life of Nietzsche now agree that Elisabeth falsified many aspects of her brother's life to create the impressions she desired. It is ironical that in promoting the idea he suffered with strokes, she gave support to the belief he was a victim of syphilis, something she indignantly denied throughout her life.

Those who work with mental patients in severely regressed states know how difficult it is to make a diagnosis solely from the deteriorated picture presented by the affected individual. It is extremely difficult to distinguish between profound mental retardation, incapacitating cerebral palsy, severely regressed schizophrenic disorders, or advanced organic brain disease once an endstate of the condition has been reached and the affected person has sunk into unresponsiveness. Nietzsche's condition during his final years of life is of little value in deciding the nature of the underlying problem. Far more important are the signs and symptoms he presented early in the course of his disorder when secondary reactions had not set in to obscure the diagnosis. The evidence from this period suggests that Nietzsche first presented with a picture of manic-depressive psychosis which gave way in time to signs of chronic schizophrenia, a not unusual sequence of events. Finally, Nietzsche gradually lapsed into a severely regressed, virtually vegetative state and died of pneumonia eleven years, eight months after onset of the psychosis.

All of the information available regarding Nietzsche's condition fits a diagnosis of "endogenous" psychosis, that is, originating within his personality structure rather than being introduced by an outside agent. The healthy and pathological coexistence of thought processes, the evidence of persecutory delusions, the incoherence of speech, the manneristic grimacing, the automatic obedience, the echolalia, the verbigeration, the volitional blunting, the social withdrawal, the regression to a vegetative state are all features of a schizophrenic disorder. On the other hand, there are grave objections to the diagnosis of general paresis in spite of the magisterial pronouncements of certain German psychiatrists.[9] The preservation of exceptional cognitive abilities at a time when the psychosis was exhibiting itself, the absence of abnormal neurological signs assignable to general paresis, the extremely slow loss of motor abilities in spite of the explosive onset of the psychological disorder, the long duration of survival beyond any similar experiences of the time, and the dubious nature of the "attacks" attributable to paresis all argue against a diagnosis of general paresis. The crucial confirmatory laboratory tests were not available and a postmortem examination was not performed. A final diagnosis of chronic schizophrenic disorder, however, is perfectly compatible with all of the manifestations of mental disorder and physical dysfunction exhibited by Nietzsche.

The concept of causation in schizophrenia at the present time is founded on the idea of an underlying "vulnerability" which puts the person at risk for the disorder. Nietzsche exhibited many of the risk factors that have been found to be associated with schizophrenic disorders. He was unmarried, he lived alone, he had no friends in his immediate surroundings, he lived in an unfamiliar environment, and possessed an inadequate grasp of the spoken language. His mode of thought was idiosyncratic to an extreme. Additionally, he had a severe visual handicap that is also a risk factor in late-onset schizophrenia.[10] His near blindness must have significantly reduced his social contacts, thus increasing his isolation. Overbeck, who knew him best, commented that his whole life was a preparation for madness.

Could Nietzsche himself have initiated his own mental disorder? All of the evidence from his writings indicating his preoccupation with madness, farce, and dissimulation make such a question necessary to consider. His closest friends, Franz Overbeck and Peter Gast, wondered about the possibility as has been discussed in Chapter 7. The pressures of his circumstances prior to his breakdown must have been intense; his inability to obtain translators which he thought to be essential for his most important works, impending financial insolvency, a public break with his mother and sister—all these factors must have created the most severe strains on his personality, especially considering his euphoric surface behavior. Perhaps he felt the state of madness was easier for him to sustain than to struggle to maintain links with an oppressive real world. Like Robert Louis Stevenson's Dr. Jekyll who could no longer escape from Mr. Hyde, perhaps Nietzsche lost the ability to return to his old condition in which he had struggled so hard to maintain himself. All this is speculation but not more speculative than the medical diagnoses that have been attached to his persona.

One may wonder, after such a far-ranging discussion, whether it makes any difference if Nietzsche suffered with general paresis, chronic schizophrenia, or some type of unique dissimulatory state. He broke down at age 44, never returned to his former creative state of mind, and died in an extremely regressed condition. Is it of any importance to try to comprehend the specifics of his mental illness? Long ago, one of his most sympathetic biographers, Charles Andler, refused to involve himself with such issues, saying that "his sloughed-off remains, consumed by an interior fire, belongs only to the psychiatrists."[11] Everything of interest about Nietzsche as a thinker and as a personality occurred prior to the breakdown of January 1889.

I submit that it is of the greatest importance to try to understand what happened to Nietzsche. If he had been an unlucky victim of paresis, it would mean that he was overcome by an external event, an invasion of his brain by the spirochetes that had entered his body years earlier. It would be an *exogenous* disorder, something coming from without which affected his mental functions. Commentators on his writings who have accepted this diagnosis have used it either to cast doubt on his ideas—for example, Möbius—or to regard it as a disinhibiting factor responsible for his creativity—for example, Lange-Eichbaum. In either case, it was an acquired disease that put the stamp on Nietzsche's thought; his ideas were a consequence of general paresis. It is the fact that Nietzsche was a paretic that needs to be remembered.

However, the diagnosis of schizophrenia casts a totally different light on the situation. Almost a century after Eugen Bleuler first coined the term, it still remains a descriptive diagnosis. Its causation is still an open question. Genetic, biochemical, psychosocial, and environmental factors are still being debated. For many years, dating back to the time of Alzheimer, changes have been described in the brains of schizophrenics subjected to neuropathological study.[12] Some degree of cortical atrophy in some schizophrenics often has been reported. More recently, complex technologies such as PET scans (positron emitted tomography) and MRI imaging (magnetic resonance imaging) have hyperdramatized metabolic and structural differences in the brains of schizophrenics.[13] None of these studies have produced a persuasive explanation of the cause of schizophrenia; the basic underlying problem of what is cause and what is correlate has not been solved. Furthermore, the fact that psychotropic medications affect the course of the disease does not mean its origin is biochemical in nature. Just as the sedative power of antianxiety drugs does not reveal the origin of anxiety, so efficacy of antipsychotic drugs does not in itself reveal the origin of schizophrenia.[14] The most judicious view is that certain individuals possess a constitutional *vulnerability* that puts them at risk for developing a schizophrenic disorder. What this "vulnerability" may be is still a mystery.

Some psychiatrists interested in Nietzsche's case rejected the diagnosis of schizophrenia because they thought it did not explain anything; for example, Ziehen and Jaspers. In a way, they were right; the diagnosis does not explain anything. It was more desirable to identify a specific etiological agent in the tradition of scientific neurology and psychiatry. But nothing is gained if the diagnosis is incorrect. Schizophrenia leaves open all possibilities and does not divert attention away from Nietzsche's mind and "the interior fire which consumed it," no matter how one interprets that fine Gallic phrase. Corman, previously quoted, has brought an existential perspective to Nietzsche's breakdown, suggesting that Nietzsche's madness was the natural consequence of the extreme nervous tension in which he lived. This view seems to bring a more insightful perspective to bear on his mental disorder. Still, it must be admitted that Nietzsche's sudden breakdown with his subsequent irreversible deterioration remains an enigma. A convincing explanation is yet to be produced as to why he descended so quickly from the heights of creative activity to a state of utter mental helplessness.

13

Nietzsche's Legacy

There is a long precedent that those who have commented on Nietzsche's health problems also concern themselves with his fundamental meaning to society. Möbius, Hildebrandt, Benda, Jaspers, and Lange-Eichbaum, for example, are writers who fall into this category. This chapter will move beyond the confines of the legend of Nietzsche's syphilis and the question of the diagnosis of his mental disorder into the broader subject of his legacy to those interested in his life and writings. There is no question that he has left a large legacy to the literate world; the nature of this legacy, however, has remained open to many different interpretations.

Nietzsche's original impact, in spite of his professions of contempt toward his native land, was mainly felt in the German-speaking world. Almost immediately after his breakdown, he began to become popular in Germanic countries. Steven Aschheim has documented the explosion of Nietzsche-consciousness at almost all levels of German society.[1] Although opinions about Nietzsche greatly varied, by and large he served to stimulate a sense of the superiority of German culture and the destiny of Germany to achieve world superiority. The rest of Europe was aware of Nietzsche's influence; according to Aschheim, a London bookseller soon after the outbreak of the First World War dubbed it the Euro-Nietzschean War.[2] Clemens Benda described from his own experience how German soldiers carried *Also Sprach Zarathustra* in their knapsacks as they marched to war.[3] The list of German writers and intellectuals who have been deeply influenced by him reads like a *Who's Who* of twentieth-century culture: Heidegger, Jaspers, Freud, Adler, Jung, Max Weber, Thomas Mann, Hermann Hesse, and Rainer Maria Rilke are only some of the names that might be mentioned.

The political passions separating Germany from most of its neighbors did not prevent Nietzsche's influence from spreading throughout Europe, especially into France. Gide, Malraux, Camus, Derrida, and Foucault are a few of the French writers of distinction who have been importantly affected by Nietzsche. Charles Andler's biography, *Nietzsche, Sa Vie et Sa Pensée*, still the most comprehensive account of the influences upon Nietzsche's intellectual development, contains a moving dedication to the memory of his students and colleagues who fell in the Great War. As might be expected, Nietzsche's influence in France has been more in the realm of philosophical concepts than in ideals wedded to the destiny of the German people.

During the interwar period, Nietzsche's writings exercised a significant influence on the theoreticians of National Socialism. The influence of the *Nietzsche Archiv*, sponsored by Elisabeth Förster-Nietzsche, was probably more significant than the writings of Nietzsche himself. Actually, the Nazi thinkers who penetrated into his works became suspicious about him and questioned his suitability as a member of the Nazi pantheon of heroes. This story is given in fascinating detail in Aschheim's chapter, "Nietzsche and the Third Reich." But for the world at large, Nietzsche was still the embodiment of German aggression and immorality. This association has never disappeared; even in Germany the feeling that somehow Nietzsche provided the philosophical groundwork of Hitlerism has remained. In 1981, an issue of *Der Spiegel* carried a cover page with a gun-wielding Hitler back to back with a reflective Nietzsche. The subscript read: "Perpetrator Hitler, Thinker Nietzsche." In spite of this association, Nietzsche has retained his place as one of the most significant figures of European thought, more so now perhaps, than ever before.

In the past, the attitude in the English-speaking world toward Nietzsche has been suspicious, generally regarding him as an early manifestation of the Germanic aggressiveness that resulted in two world wars. This belief has radically changed in recent decades. Now instead of only a small circle of professional philologists and philosophers, there is a wave of interest in Nietzsche at many levels in the United States and Great Britain. In the last ten years, there have been over 250 English-language books published dealing with Nietzsche, more than have appeared in German-reading countries. A casual survey of philosophy sections in major book stores will usually reveal more books on Nietzsche than on any other literary figure. Nietzsche has achieved popularity in English-speaking countries, a state of affairs once only dreamed of by Nietzsche himself.

To what can Nietzsche's continual and pervasive interest be attributed? He has often been described as a master of German prose style but he is rarely read because of his stylistic brilliance. Furthermore, although the excellence of style does not easily translate into other languages, particularly into English, he has become at least as much an object of interest in English-speaking countries as in his native Germany. His philosophical positions are hardly those which would secure him such international popularity. The ideas he worked out, often spottily and with internal contradictions; for example, *amor fati* (love one's fate), the idea of eternal recurrence, the relativity of values, Christianity as the *bête noire* of European civilization, aristocratic radicalism—the ultimate political incorrectness—are hardly those which would command him a wide audience. He laughed at the principal metaphysical dogma of Western civilization—belief in God—and went a step beyond Heine in sarcasm by saying God was not only made sick by man but had died of grief over his condition. He would have nothing to do with ideas such as immortality, separateness of soul or any kind of special revelation. But he was no more entranced with the mechanistic theories of science which he saw as manifestations of limited and self-serving minds. Socialists and anarchists he viewed as ridiculous *canaille*. He thought compassion to be the principal danger for the developed human being; contempt being his natural state of mind. His comments about women are best left unrepeated. For all these reasons, he has been regarded as the ultimate nihilist of European culture. Nihilism is rarely a point of view that attracts many adherents.

Then why is Nietzsche so popular? I submit it is because he

projects his commitment to the primacy of the individual and stands for the freedom of his potential. All the cultural traditions within which individuals are so prone to become entangled are relegated to the category of traps for the unwary. When reading Nietzsche, one feels oneself to be in the presence of someone who, by speaking for himself, speaks for independently-minded individuals the world over. There is an enormous difference in reading Nietzsche as compared to reading about him. All the scholarly commentators who analyze his work give their literary judgments within the context of scholarly analysis. But Nietzsche reveals his inner self while still retaining his intellectual conscience. He creates his own special world in the tension, as phrased by Walter Kaufmann, between analysis and existentialism.[4] His thoughts, his intuitions, his dislikes, and his positive passions are all personal. We feel in experiencing his *Geist*[5] that we are making contact with an individual who has risen above the institutional trappings of his society and wishes to communicate his perspectives to the reader. Such an author is very rare.

His influence must be placed within the framework of a radical mental individualism; outwardly he may have been a modest retired professor but inwardly he was a revolutionary thinker, his works were dynamite as was noted by a perceptive reviewer prior to his achieving fame.[6] One could think that Emerson was anticipating Nietzsche when he wrote: "Beware when the great God lets loose a thinker on this planet. Then all things are at risk. It is as when a conflagration has broken out in a great city, and no man knows what is safe, or where it will end. . . ."[7] This is why Nietzsche often has been deemed unsafe for "immature" minds. In fact, he is unsafe reading for all minds if by unsafe one means that the conventional channels of one's life may be disrupted and the individual himself put at risk.

A casual inspection of almost any part of Nietzsche's works immediately reveals that one is in the presence of a writer of great originality of both thought and style. His masks were meant to be seen through by discriminating readers, his hyperbole was meant to shake them free of ossified habits of thinking. His purpose was not to divert his audience but to elevate them—if the will to elevation were present. Once one becomes accustomed to his style, his jokes, exaggerations, and sarcasms, the reader becomes aware of someone, as Nietzsche himself said of Schopenhauer, "whose power and well-being envelop us from the first sound of his voice; we feel as we do when we enter an Alpine forest, we take a deep breath and suddenly feel better."[8] It is an excellent recommendation for a writer to say he is not for immature minds, since adult readers should not want to read what is suitable for the immature. One feels that Nietzsche uninhibitedly speaks the truth as he has understood it through the perspective of his experience of life. What else can be expected of any philosopher?

Anyone who discusses Nietzsche needs to quote him often and at length because the essential points come only from the writings of Nietzsche himself. He expresses himself, not as a scholar or critic, but from the vantage-point of his own individuality; thus his tone is original and incapable of duplication by others. There are few who surpass him in familiarity with the history of culture but this is not the focus of his efforts. He writes as one individual to another—to those others who are open to his ideas—which is a very different matter from scholarly or didactic communication. Any style was good, he said, which genuinely communicated an inward state. For example, consider this extract from the forward to *Ecce Homo, s.* 3, written by Nietzsche at a time when spirochetes were supposed to be destroying his brain:

Whoever knows how to breathe the air of my writings knows that it is an air of heights, a *strong* air. One must be made for it, otherwise there is no small danger to become chilled by it. The ice is near, the solitude is immense—but how calm lies everything in the light! How free one breathes! How much one feels to be *below* oneself! Philosophy, as I have until now understood it and lived it, is the voluntary life in ice and high mountains—the seeking-out of everything strange and questionable in existence, everything which up to now has been banned by morality. From long experience with such wandering in the *forbidden*, I discovered that the fundamental causes, which up to now have given rise to moralizing and idealizing, seem very different than might be expected: the *concealed* history of the philosophers, of the great names of psychology, was revealed to me. How much truth can a mind *endure*, how much truth can it *dare*? Increasingly for me, that has become the real measure of value. Error (faith in an ideal) is not blindness, error is *cowardice* . . . every accomplishment, every step forward in knowledge *follows* from courage, from strength in oneself, from purity towards oneself . . . I don't oppose ideals, I merely put on gloves before them. *Nitimur in vetitum* [we strive for the forbidden—Ovid]: with this thought my philosophy will conquer one day because what has been forbidden has always been only the truth.

Whoever does not have a sense for metaphysical thought will never appreciate Nietzsche. Scholars who are steeped in the analytical materialism of the times find no common ground with him no matter how much they may acquire expertise on his life and the content of his writings. He himself opposed the "metaphysical need" of people, having heavily attacked the principal metaphysical ideal of European culture; that is, Christianity and the tenets connected with it. But this was because Nietzsche had his own metaphysical ideal that he set above all those of his society. This ideal was the free human spirit, the striving individual self which creates all values. Reality was to be found in this self, not in the surface activities and impersonal values he experienced in his society. He states this ideal most clearly in *Beyond Good and Evil* (s. 287):

What is noble? What does the word "noble" (*vornehm*) mean to us today? What reveals itself, how can one recognize the noble person under the densely overcast sky of mob rule, by virtue of which everything becomes opaque and leaden? It is not his actions which prove him, actions are always ambiguous, always hard to evaluate; neither is it his "works." One finds today, among artists and scholars, many whose works reveal how deeply they desire to be noble: however just this need to be noble is basically different from the needs of the noble soul itself, actually the eloquent and dangerous sign of its lack. It is not deeds, it is *faith* which is decisive here, which here determines a hierarchy—to take up again an old religious formula in a newer and deeper sense. It is some kind of fundamental knowledge that a noble soul has about itself, something which cannot be sought, cannot be found and perhaps cannot be lost. *The noble soul has reverence for itself.*

These words sound strange to the modern mind. The enlightened individual today has persuaded himself that there is no such thing as a soul or a spirit. There is only a brain with a hundred billion nerve cells, intricately wired together, creating a vast network of electrical activity which is the physical reality behind such illusory concepts as soul or spirit. The model to be studied is the mighty computer which accomplishes all things, not the archaic concepts of bygone days. Nietzsche himself did not take this biological materialism very seriously. Religious superstitions, not scientific dogmas, were the main obstacles he saw to enlightenment of the spirit for those who were capable of achieving it. But he lived at a time of great expansion of scientific activity and occasionally he expressed himself on the subject. The following is from *The Gay Science* (s. 373):

"Science" as Bias. It follows from the laws of hierarchy, that scholars, insofar as they belong to a spiritual middle class, cannot envisage the really *important* problems and question marks; their courage or their vision do not reach that far. Above all, their needs which made them into researchers, their inner desires and presuppositions that things should exist in *such and such* a manner, their fears and hopes too quickly come to rest and are satisfied. It is the same thing with the faith with which so many materialistic natural scientists are satisfied, the faith in a world that has its equivalents and measures in human thinking and human valuations, in a "world of truth" at which one arrives at last with the help of our square little human reason. What? Do we really want to degrade our existence into a computerized servitude and grubbing about of mathematicians? Above all, one should not want to deprive it of its *many-sided* character: but that requires *good* taste, gentlemen, above all, a taste for reverence of that which lies beyond your horizons! That the only interpretation of the world should be just the one which is your interpretation, in which scientific study can proceed in *your* sense (do you really mean *mechanistically?*) in which is permitted only counting, calculating, weighing, seeing and touching and nothing more; that is crudity and naiveté, if it is not mental disease or imbecility. Would it not be more probable that just this most superficial and external aspect of existence—the most visible, its skin and sensory part—is the first to be grasped? Perhaps the only one to be grasped? A "scientific" interpretation of the world, as you understand it, would consequently be one of the most *slow-witted*, meaning the most impoverished, of all possible interpretations of the world: this is said into the ear and conscience of those mechanists who today run about among philosophers and think that mechanics provide the exclusive laws on which the foundation of all existence must be based. But an essentially mechanical world would be an essentially *meaningless* world! Assuming that one could determine the value of a piece of music according to how one counts, calculates and makes formulas of it—how absurd such a "scientific" determination of music would be! What would have one grasped, understood, recognized about it! Nothing, exactly nothing of what "music" really is!

Nietzsche lived his life prior to his breakdown according to his ideas and his values. His separation from the institutions of his time permitted him to live a free interior life. He was willing to wait for the readers who finally did come—although not until after he could no longer be aware of them. Externally, there were no events in his life of distinction, his was the inconspicuous existence of a retired professor with a small pension. He had no significant known vices nor did he behave in any manner that would arouse attention until psychosis overcame him. It was only his thoughts which distinguished him, the thoughts which he scribbled down in his letters, notebooks, and manuscripts. He said that the greatest thoughts *were* the greatest events;[9] western society has come to agree with him since his memory towers far above the movers and shakers of his era who have been largely relegated to the history books. He can be compared to individuals like Thoreau and Kierkegaard who also lived outside the institutions of their time, who also made little impact on their contemporaries but whose thoughts have also become the great events of the world.

One should not make an idol of Nietzsche nor did he wish to become one. He had many character faults; at times, he could be boastful, deceitful, resentful and self-pitying. *Amor fati* for him was a goal to be sought, not a part of his normal temper. Henry David Thoreau, whose life and thoughts have many similarities to Nietzsche's, possessed a far more integrated personality. Ultimately the discrepancies between Nietzsche's ideals and the realities of his psychic structure became so great that he collapsed into psychosis. He should not be regarded as a martyr but as a human being whose personal capacities could not keep pace with his aspirations. He is more Icarus than Jesus Christ, his life proves that there are limits to one's ability to create oneself and that the art of living consists in discovering these limits, not prematurely, not out of a feeling of fear or an inordinate desire for the goods of society, but out of a realistic sense of one's own capacities to fulfill self-imposed tasks. Nietzsche was given good advice by Strindberg in the latter's last letter to him, unfortunately, it came too late in the day to be of use.

The popularity of Nietzsche in America may have a certain national basis not existing elsewhere. There are considerable similarities between Bismarckian Germany of his day, the "Second

Reich," and the United States at the end of the twentieth century. Both were the national powerhouses of their time, both exerted a hegemonial influence which was based on economic and military power. Bismarck's Germany based its national pride on the concept of German "Kultur"; today, in the United States, it is technological mastery that is the touchstone of its self-confidence. In either case, the consequences were an enormous development of the power of institutional structures within the countries and a corresponding diminishment of the capacity of the individual to develop himself as an independent entity. Nietzsche may have been an expatriate, but he lived under the shadow of the values of German cultural institutions. Referring to the triumph of Germany over France in the 1870 war, Nietzsche commented that the victory of the German Reich led to the extinction of the German spirit.[10] Some such process may be afoot today in the United States. Its economic and scientific hegemony creates institutions of such power that the free spirit of the individual can hardly breathe. The materialist orientation is preeminent and dominates the life of individuals whatever their profession or way of life.

Henry David Thoreau wrote in the first chapter of *Walden* (1854) that the mass of men lived lives of quiet desperation. It is unlikely his judgment would be any different today. Perhaps this is why so many individuals resonate sympathetically to the thoughts expressed by Nietzsche whose desperate state was not very quiet. Of course, there are not many who suffer as much as Nietzsche did, just as there are few who possess his genius, insight, and capacity for self-expression. But the issues of his day are still the issues of our day. The focus of our society is on the "ideals" of self-serving participants in a system which, more and more, is being felt to be a latter-day Roman Empire imposing its values on all the world. But in the long run, the only really significant factor in human society as was asserted by Max Weber, founder of scientific sociology, is the free, *value-creating* initiative of the individual personality.[11] That is why interest in Nietzsche persists and his legacy lives on today. But his should be the last voice on this subject; herein follows one of the final passages of *Ecce Homo* (Why I Am a Destiny, s.1) which reveals simultaneously his vision, his insight, his hubris and the disregard of societal reality which led to his breakdown (Why I Am a Destiny, s.1):

I know my fate. Someday something tremendous will be connected with my name—a crisis as has never before been on the earth, the profoundest crisis of conscience, a decision *against* everything which had been heretofore believed, required, made holy. I am not a man, I am dynamite. Yet with all that, there is nothing within me to found a religion—religions are mob affairs, I find it necessary to wash my hands after contact with religious people . . . I *don't want* any "believers." I think I am too malicious to believe even in myself and I never speak to mobs . . . I have a terrifying feeling that one day I will be called holy; this is why I have brought forth this book *before*, it will prevent people from talking nonsense about me . . . I am no saint, I would rather be a clown . . . perhaps I am a clown . . . but in spite of this or rather not in spite of this—since up to now nobody has lied more than saints—the truth speaks out from me. My truth is *frightening* since heretofore, lies have been called truth. *Transformation of all Values*: that is my formula for an act of supreme self-consciousness of humanity that has become flesh and genius in me. My fate is that I must be the first *upright* person, that I know myself to be in opposition to the lies of thousands of years . . . I am the first to have *discovered* the truth by means of seeing lies as lies, *smelling* them . . . my genius is in my nostrils . . . I oppose as has never been opposed before, and, in spite of this, I am not a nay-saying spirit. I bring *glad tidings* such as have never been brought before, I know tasks of such enormity as have never been envisaged; I am the first to again give hope. With all this, I am necessarily also a calamitous person. For when the truth enters into conflict with the lies of millennia, there will be upheavals, the convulsions of earthquakes, the movement of mountains and valleys, the like of which has never been dreamt of before. The concept of politics will then be given up in a spiritual war, all the powers of the old society will evaporate into thin air—they are based entirely on lies: there will be strife such as has never been before. I am the first to bring to the world *great politics*.[12]

Notes

PREFACE

1. Anacleto Verrecchia, *Zarathustra's Ende* (Vienna: Böhlaus, 1986) (originally, *La Catastrophe di Nietzsche a Torino*, 1976).
2. Paul Julius Möbius, *Über das Pathologische bei Nietzsche* (Wiesbaden: Bergmann, 1902).
3. Pia Daniela Volz, *Nietzsche im Labyrinth Seiner Krankheit* (Würzburg: Königshausen and Neumann, 1990).
4. Walter Harding and Carl Bode, eds., *The Correspondence of Henry David Thoreau* (New York: New York University Press, 1958), 265.
5. Verrecchia, 326.

CHAPTER 1

1. Janz, however, notes that there is reason to believe Nietzsche was distantly related to Goethe, the Schlegel brothers and—most surprisingly!—Richard Wagner. Curt Paul Janz, *Friedrich Nietzsche, Biographie*, 3 volumes, 2d ed. (Munich: Carl Hanser, 1993), Vol. 1, 32.
2. Janz, Vol. 3, 173.
3. Janz, Vol. 1, 34.
4. Janz, Vol. 1, 46.
5. Möbius, 10–11.
6. Janz, Vol. 2, 77.

CHAPTER 2

1. Janz, Vol. 1, 52.
2. Janz, Vol. 1, 62.
3. Volz, 92.
4. Ronald Hayman, *Nietzsche, a Critical Life* (New York: Oxford University Press, 1980), 27–28.
5. Janz, Vol. 1, 128–129.

CHAPTER 3

1. Hayman, 61.
2. Janz, Vol. 1, 136–137.
3. Janz, Vol. 1, 137–138.
4. Volz, 190.
5. Janz, Vol. 1, 161.
6. Kurt Hildebrandt, *Gesundheit und Krankheit in Nietzsches Leben und Werk* (Berlin: Karger, 1926), 108.
7. Wilhelm Lange-Eichbaum, *Nietzsche, Krankheit und Wirkung* (Hamburg: Anton Lettenbauer, 1948).
8. Volz, 190–191.

CHAPTER 4

1. Hayman, 129.
2. Hildebrandt, 112.
3. Hayman, 143.
4. Volz, 317–323.
5. Walter Kaufmann, *Nietzsche, Philosopher, Psychologist, Antichrist*, 4th ed. (Princeton: Princeton University Press, 1974), 8.
6. Volz, 340–343.
7. Volz, 345–349.
8. Richard Schain, *Philosophical Artwork* (Glen Ellen, CA: Garric Press, 1983), 47.

CHAPTER 5

1. Janz, Vol. 2, 257.
2. Janz, Vol. 2, 271.
3. Volz, 163.
4. Stefan Zweig, *Baumeister der Welt* (Frankfurt: S. Fischer, 1951), 309–311.
5. Hayman, 361.

6. Lange-Eichbaum, 88.

7. Lesley Chamberlain, *Nietzsche in Turin* (New York: Picador, 1996), 200–201.

8. David F. Krell and Donald L. Bates, *The Good European* (Chicago: University of Chicago, 1997), 47.

CHAPTER 6

1. R. J. Hollingdale, *Nietzsche* (London: Ark, 1985), 238.

2. Walter Kaufmann, *The Portable Nietzsche* (New York: Viking, 1954), 568.

3. Raoul Richter, in *Nietzsche Ecce Homo* (Frankfurt: Insel Verlag, 1979), 24.

4. Verrecchia, 234ff.

5. Verrecchia, 273.

6. Verrecchia, 266ff.

7. Verrecchia, 255.

8. Verrecchia, 265.

9. Oscar Levy, ed., *Selected Letters of Friedrich Nietzsche* (Garden City, NY: Doubleday, 1921), 311.

CHAPTER 7

1. Janz, Vol. 3, 50.

2. Volz, 380–381.

3. Volz, 384.

4. Verrecchia, 329.

5. Janz, Vol. 3, 82.

6. Volz, 386–387.

7. Volz, 533–534.

8. Volz, 392–393.

9. "The impression that a conspicuous scar means a previous chancre is a widespread error." J.H. Stokes, H. Beerman, and N.R. Ingrahay, *Modern Clinical Syphilology*, 3rd ed. (Philadelphia: Saunders, 1944), 479.

10. Volz, 390–415.

11. Volz, 400.

12. Volz, 405.

13. Janz, Vol. 3, 103.

14. E. F. Podach, *The Madness of Nietzsche* (London: Putnam, 1931), 213.

15. Podach, 214.

16. Podach, 215.

17. Podach, 217.

18. Podach, 225.

19. *Ecce Homo*, Why I Am So Wise (s.3). Older editions usually contain the earlier version that was preferred by Kaufmann.

20. Michael Gelder, Dennis Gath, and Richard Mayou, *Oxford Textbook of Psychiatry*, 2nd ed. (Oxford: Oxford University Press, 1989), 312–313.

CHAPTER 8

1. Hayman, 342–343.
2. Hayman, 345.
3. Verrecchia, 343.
4. Elisabeth had married Bernhard Förster, an advocate of traditional German virtues free of Jewish influences. Nietzsche intensely disliked most professional antisemites, including his new brother-in-law. When Förster's venture in Paraguay collapsed, he committed suicide. The angry colonists demanded that Elisabeth leave, having experienced her as a disruptive and mendacious influence. See H.F. Peters, *Zarathustra's Sister* (New York: Markus Wiener, 1977).
5. Sandor Gilman, *Conversations with Nietzsche* (New York: Oxford University Press, 1987), 254–255.
6. Volz, 496.
7. Hayman, 350.
8. Volz, 533.
9. Volz, 234.
10. Friedrich Würzbach, *Nietzsche* (Berlin: Propyläen Verlag, 1942), 427.
11. J. Fuchs, "Friedrich Nietzsches Augenleiden," *Münchner Medizinische Wochenschrift* 120 (1978): 631–634.
12. Möbius, 102.

CHAPTER 9

1. Frederick C. Redlich and Daniel X. Freedman, *The Theory and Practice of Psychiatry* (New York: Basic Books, 1966), 35.
2. In Emil Kraepelin, *Psychiatrie*, 5th ed. (Leipzig: Barth, 1896), 541.
3. E. H. Hare, "Origin and Spread of Dementia Paralytica," *Journal of Mental Science* 105 (1959): 594–626.
4. Emil Kraepelin, *"General Paresis*, Monograph Section 14," *Journal of Nervous and Mental Diseases* 63 (1913): 209.
5. S.A. Kinnier Wilson, *Neurology*, Vol. 1 (New York: Hafner, 1940), 51.
6. Kraeplin, *"General Paresis,"* 209.
7. Kraepelin, *Psychiatrie*, 515.
8. Wilson, 532.

9. Volz, 444.

10. Kraepelin, *Psychiatrie*, 471–472.

11. Karl Kleist, "Die Gegenwärtigen Stromungen in der Psychiatrie," *Zeitschrift für Psychiatrie* 82 (1925): 1–41.

12. Wilhelm Zeh, *Progressive Paralyse* (Stuttgart: Thieme, 1964).

13. Zeh, 102.

14. A. Risse, A. Rohde, and A. Marneros, "Erscheinungsformen der Progressiven Paralyse," *Deutsche Medizinische Wochenschrift* 110 (1985): 1202–1205.

15. Zeh, 1.

16. Volz, 447–448.

17. Kraepelin, *Psychiatrie*, 426–471.

18. Heinz E. Lehmann, "Schizophrenia: Clinical Features." In *Comprehensive Textbook of Psychiatry*, Vol. 2, Harold I. Kaplan, Alfred M. Freedman, and Benjamin J. Saddock, eds. (Baltimore: Williams & Wilkins, 1980), 1156.

19. Kraepelin, *Psychiatrie*, 434.

20. A.J. Saykin et al., "Neuropsychological Function in Schizophrenia," *Archives of General Psychiatry* 48 (1991): 618–624.

21. Kurt Goldstein, "The Significance of Special Mental Tests for Diagnosis and Prognosis in Schizophrenia," *American Journal of Psychiatry* 96 (1939): 575–588.

22. Redlich and Freedman, 478.

CHAPTER 10

1. Max Nordau, *Degeneration* (New York: D. Appleton & Co., 1895).

2. Emil Kraepelin, *Einführung in die Psychiatrische Klinik* (Leipzig: J. A. Barth, 1916). 3rd ed.

3. Hildebrandt, 156.

4. Hildebrandt, 158.

5. E. F. Podach, *Nietzsches Zusammenbruch* (Heidelberg: Niels Kampmann, 1930).

6. Many of the significant comments in the appendices are not found in the previously cited English translation (*Madness of Nietzsche*).

7. Karl Jaspers, *Nietzsche* (Tucson: University of Arizona Press, 1966), 89.

8. Jaspers, 100.

9. Jaspers, 97.

10. Kurt Kolle, "Nietzsche, Krankheit und Werk," *Aktuelle Fragen der Psychiatrie und Neurologie* 2 (1965): 106–121.

11. Verrecchia, 326.

12. Ernst Benda [C.E. Benda], "Nietzsche's Krankheit," *Monatschrift für Psychiatrie und Neurologie*, 60 (1925): 65–80.

13. Clemens E. Benda, "Über die Krankheit Friedrich Nietzsches," *Medizinische Welt* 17 (1965): 951–959, 1013–1018.

14. Wilson, 533.

15. H. Houston Merritt, Raymond D. Adams, and Harry C. Solomon, *Neurosyphilis* (New York: Oxford University Press, 1946), 222.

16. Zeh, 102.

17. Wilson, 562.

18. Louis Corman, *Nietzsche, Psychologue des Profondeurs* (Paris: Presses Universitaires, 1982), 409–410.

19. Volz, 298.

20. Volz's book is based on her doctoral dissertation for the University of Tübingen. Supposedly, the medical faculty of the university opposed her conclusion. John Banville, Letter to the Editor, "Nietzsche's Complaint," *New York Review of Books*, November 5, 1998, 62.

CHAPTER 11

1. Fuchs, 631.

2. Volz, 92.

3. Volz, 90–118.

4. Volz, 110.

5. Volz, 347.

6. Daniel. G. Vaughn, Taylor Asbury, and Paul Riordan-Eva, *General Ophthalmology*, 14th ed. (Norwalk, Conn.: Appleton-Lange, 1995), 192.

7. Light sensitivity was a recurrent problem for Nietzsche in sunny southern Europe which he otherwise preferred. He tried to use special lenses to protect his eyes but the difficulty with sunlight is frequently mentioned in his letters.

8. Volz, 105.

CHAPTER 12

1. Redlich and Freedman, 548.

2. *Diagnostic and Statistical Manual of Mental Disorders, DSM-IV* (Washington: American Psychiatric Association, 1994), 292–296.

3. Volz, 481.

4. Volz, 487.

5. Volz, 488ff.

6. Since Nietzsche was right-handed (Gilman, 247, 253), an attack leaving him speechless would be expected to involve the right side of his body.

7. Volz, 503.

8. Paul Möbius asserted in the foreword of the 2d edition of his monograph on Nietzsche that the death mask revealed an asymmetry indicating facial paralysis. Physicians who try to interpret facial asymmetries know how difficult it can be draw conclusions except in obvious cases. In Nietzsche's life, facial paralysis was not noted.

9. Ziehen was still saying in 1938 that the course of Nietzsche's illness "left no doubt" that it was syphilitic in origin. Sander L. Gilman, "Friedrich Nietzsche's Conversation Notebooks," B. Urban and W. Kudzus eds., *Psychoanalytische und Psychopathologische Literaturinterpretation* (Darmstadt: Wissenschaftliche Buchgesellschaft, 1981), 338.

10. Godfrey Pearlson and Peter Rabins, "Late-onset Psychoses, Possible Risk Factors," *Psychiatric Clinics of North America* 11 (1988): 15–32.

11. Charles Andler, *Nietzsche, Sa Vie et Sa Pensée*, Vol. 2 (Paris: Gallimard, 1958), 260 (first published 1920).

12. Raymond D. Adams and Maurice Victor, *Principles of Neurology*, 5th ed. (New York: McGraw-Hill, 1993), 1335–1336.

13. Jonathan D. Brodie, "Imaging for the Clinical Psychiatrist," *American Journal of Psychiatry* 153 (1996): 145–149.

14. Overactivity of the pathways of the neurotransmitter dopamine has been widely speculated to be the underlying physiological fault in schizophrenia. However, evidence that there is an underlying defect in schizophrenics involving dopamine has not been forthcoming, even though there is much data indicating that antipsychotic drugs exert their effects through blocking dopamine metabolism.

CHAPTER 13

1. Steven E. Aschheim, *The Nietzsche Legacy in Germany 1890–1990* (Berkeley: University of California, 1992).

2. Aschheim, 128.

3. Benda, 1965, 953.

4. Walter Kaufmann, *Existentialism from Dostoevsky to Sartre* (New York: Meridian, 1975), 51 (first published 1956).

5. It is well known that there is no English word which adequately conveys the full spiritual-intellectual-emotional connotation of the German word *Geist*.

6. Janz, Vol. 2, 497.

7. Ralph Waldo Emerson, *Essays: First Series*, "Circles," Brooks Atkinson, ed. (New York: Random House, 1940), 283.

8. *Schopenhauer as Educator* (s.2).

9. *Beyond Good and Evil* (s.285).

10. *David Strauss Confessor and Writer* (s.1).

11. Wolfgang J. Mommsen, *The Age of Bureaucracy, Perspectives on the Political Sociology of Max Weber* (New York: Harper & Row, 1974), 98.

12. In 1900, Peter Gast ended his effusive oration at Nietzsche's gravesite by saying, "Peace on your ashes! Holy be your name to all future generations!" It was followed by singing from the male choir. Had Nietzsche been there to listen, he surely would have been laid low by a migrainous attack.

Selected Bibliography

Adams, Raymond D. and Maurice Victor. *Principles of Neurology*, 5th ed. New York: McGraw-Hill, pp. 620–627, 1993. (the contemporary approach to neurosyphilis)

Andler, Charles. *Nietzsche, Sa Vie et Sa Pensée*. Paris: Gallimard, 1958. (first published 1920)

Aschheim, Steven E. *The Nietzsche Legacy in Germany 1890–1990*. Berkeley: University of California, 1992.

Benda, Clemens E. "Über die Krankheit Friedrich Nietzsches." *Medizinische Welt* 17: 951–959, 1013–1018, 1965.

Chamberlain, Lesley. *Nietzsche in Turin*. New York: Picador, 1996.

Corman, Louis. *Nietzsche, Psychologue des Profondeurs*. Paris: Presses Universitaires, pp. 409–410, 1982.

Gilman, Sandor. *Conversations with Nietzsche*. New York: Oxford University Press, 1987.

Hayman, Ronald. *Nietzsche, a Critical Life*. New York: Oxford University Press, 1980.

Hildebrandt, Kurt. *Gesundheit und Krankheit in Nietzsches Leben und Werk*. Berlin: Karger, 1926.

Hollingdale, R.J. *Nietzsche*. London: Ark, 1985.

Janz, Curt Paul. *Friedrich Nietzsche, Biographie*, 2d ed. Munich: Carl Hanser, 1993. (the definitive biography)

Jaspers, Karl. *Nietzsche*. Tucson: University of Arizona Press, 1966.

Kaplan, H.I., Alfred M. Freedman, and Benjamin Saddock. *Comprehensive*

Textbook of Psychiatry/III. Baltimore: Williams and Wilkins, 1980. (interesting discussions of history of psychiatry in the nineteenth century)

Kaufmann, Walter. *The Portable Nietzsche*. New York: Viking, 1954.

———. *Existentialism from Dostoevsky to Sartre*. New York: Meridian, 1975. (first published 1956)

———. *Nietzsche, Philosopher, Psychologist, Antichrist*, 4th ed. Princeton: Princeton University Press, 1974.

Kolle, Kurt. "Nietzsche, Krankheit und Werk." *Aktuelle Fragen der Psychiatrie und Neurologie* 2:106–121, 1965.

Kraepelin, Emil. *Psychiatrie*, 5th ed., Leipzig: Barth, 1896. (classic clinical descriptions from institutional psychiatry in nineteenth-century Germany)

———. "General Paresis, Monograph Section 14." *Journal of Nervous and Mental Diseases* 63, 1913.

Krell, David F. and Donald L. Bates. *The Good European*. Chicago: University of Chicago, 1997.

Merritt, H. Houston, Raymond D. Adams, and Harry C. Solomon. *Neurosyphilis*. New York: Oxford University Press, 1946. (American review of illness prior to antibiotic era)

Möbius, Paul Julius. *Über das Pathologische bei Nietzsche*. Wiesbaden: Bergmann, 1902.

Peters, H.F. *Zarathustra's Sister*. New York: Markus Wiener, 1977.

Podach, E.F. *Nietzsches Zusammenbruch*. Heidelberg: Niels Kampmann, 1930.

———. *The Madness of Nietzsche*. London: Putnam, 1931.

Ross, Werner. *Der ängstliche Adler: Friedrich Nietzsche's Leben*. Stuttgart: Deutsche Verlag Anstatt, 1980.

Schiller, Francis. *A Möbius Strip. Fin-de-Siècle Neuropsychiatry and Paul Möbius*. Berkeley: University of California Press, 1982.

Verrecchia, Anacleto. *Zarathustra's Ende*. Vienna: Böhlaus, 1986. (fascinating discussion of Nietzsche's last month in Turin)

Volz, Pia Daniela. *Nietzsche im Labyrinth Seiner Krankheit*. Würzburg: Königshausen and Neumann, 1990.

Wilson, S.A.K. *Neurology*, Vol. 1. New York: Hafner, 1940. (comprehensive descriptions of neurosyphilis prior to the antibiotic era)

Würzbach, Friedrich. *Nietzsche*. Berlin: Propyläen Verlag, 1942.

Zeh, Wilhelm. *Progressive Paralyse*. Stuttgart: Thieme, 1964.

Zweig, Stefan. *Baumeister der Welt*. Frankfurt: S. Fischer, 1951.

Index

About the Author

RICHARD SCHAIN is currently a neurological consultant at a California state hospital. He was formerly Professor of Neurology and Psychiatry at the University of Nebraska and Head of the Division of Child Neurology at the University of California, Los Angeles. He has published numerous articles, chapters, and books, including *Neurology of Childhood Learning Disorders*, *Affirmations of Reality*, and *Philosophical Artwork*.

Recent Titles in
Contributions in Medical Studies

A Community Approach to AIDS Intervention: Exploring the Miami Outreach Project for Injecting Drug Users and Other High Risk Groups
Dale D. Chitwood, James A. Inciardi, Duane C. McBride, Clyde B. McCoy, H. Virginia McCoy, and Edward Trapido

Beyond Flexner: Medical Education in the Twentieth Century
Barbara Barzansky and Norman Gevitz, editors

Mother and Fetus: Changing Notions of Maternal Responsibility
Robert H. Blank

The Golden Wand of Medicine: A History of the Caduceus Symbol in Medicine
Walter J. Friedlander

Cancer Factories: America's Tragic Quest for Uranium Self-Sufficiency
Howard Ball

The AIDS Pandemic: Social Perspectives
Howard Ball

Childbed Fever: A Scientific Biography of Ignaz Semmelweis
K. Codell Carter and Barbara R. Carter

James Cook and the Conquest of Scurvy
Francis E. Cuppage

Romance, Poetry, and Surgical Sleep: Literature Influences Medicine
E. M. Papper

Sex, Disease, and Society
Milton Lewis, Scott Bamber, and M. Waugh, editors

Histories of Sexually Transmitted Diseases and HIV/AIDS in Sub-Saharan Africa
Philip W. Setal, Milton Lewis, and Maryinez Lyons, editors

The History of Modern Epilepsy: The Beginning, 1865–1914
Walter J. Friedlander